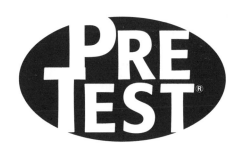

Pathophysiology

PreTest® Self-Assessment and Review

Notice

Medicine is an ever-changing science. As new research and clinical experience broaden our knowledge, changes in treatment and drug therapy are required. The authors and the publisher of this work have checked with sources believed to be reliable in their efforts to provide information that is complete and generally in accord with the standards accepted at the time of publication. However, in view of the possibility of human error or changes in medical sciences, neither the authors nor the publisher nor any other party who has been involved in the preparation or publication of this work warrants that the information contained herein is in every respect accurate or complete, and they disclaim all responsibility for any errors or omissions or for the results obtained from use of the information contained in this work. Readers are encouraged to confirm the information contained herein with other sources. For example and in particular, readers are advised to check the product information sheet included in the package of each drug they plan to administer to be certain that the information contained in this work is accurate and that changes have not been made in the recommended dose or in the contraindications for administration. This recommendation is of particular importance in connection with new or infrequently used drugs.

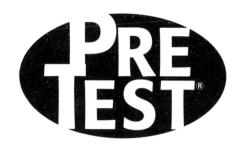

Pathophysiology
PreTest® Self-Assessment and Review
Second Edition

Maurice A. Mufson, M.D., M.A.C.P.

Professor of Medicine
Chairman Emeritus
Department of Medicine
Marshall University School of Medicine
Huntington, West Virginia

Student Reviewers

Christopher A. Heck

University of South Alabama College of Medicine
Mobile, Alabama
Class of 2001

Sara M. Nesler

University of Iowa College of Medicine
Iowa City, Iowa
Class of 2002

McGraw-Hill
Medical Publishing Division

New York   Chicago   San Francisco   Lisbon   London   Madrid   Mexico City
Milan   New Delhi   San Juan   Seoul   Singapore   Sydney   Toronto

McGraw-Hill

A Division of The **McGraw·Hill** Companies

Pathophysiology: PreTest® Self-Assessment and Review, Second Edition

1 2 3 4 5 6 7 8 9 0   DOC/DOC   0 9 8 7 6 5 4 3 2 1

ISBN 0-07-137507-4

This book was set in Berkeley by North Market Street Graphics.
The editor was Catherine A. Johnson.
The production supervisor was Phil Galea.
Project management was provided by North Market Street Graphics.
The cover designer was Li Chen Chang / Pinpoint.
R.R. Donnelley & Sons was printer and binder.

This book is printed on acid-free paper.

Cataloging-in-Publication data is on file for this title at the Library of Congress.

Contents

Gastroenterology

Liver Disease

Thyroid and Pituitary Disorders

Reproductive System

Nervous System

Contributors

Shirley M. Neitch, M.D.

Professor of Medicine
Section Chief of Geriatrics
Department of Medicine
Marshall University School of Medicine
Huntington, West Virginia

Henry K. Driscoll, M.D.

Professor of Medicine
Department of Medicine
Marshall University School of Medicine
Huntington, West Virginia

Jason Yap, M.D.

Assistant Professor of Medicine
Section Chief of Nephrology
Department of Medicine
Marshall University School of Medicine
Huntington, West Virginia

Paulette Wehner, M.D.

Associate Professor of Medicine
Director of Cardiology Fellowship
Department of Cardiovascular Services
Marshall University School of Medicine
Huntington, West Virginia

Introduction

Testing your knowledge by answering the pathophysiology questions in this book serves as a competition in which you compete against yourself for the satisfaction of doing well. It's a great feeling when you know the answers to difficult medical questions. It reflects well on your ability to learn the material in medical school, and it's a signal that you're prepared for the certifying examinations. This competition also can increase your knowledge base, as any competition sharpens your skills. That is an important part of testing ourselves. When we don't know an answer, it's an opportunity to look it up in a "big book" of internal medicine and improve our understanding of the topic. Each answer includes a reference to that answer, as a starting point for reading more about the topic. Although knowing the answer to any individual question provides some measure of satisfaction, it does not, and should not, represent a stopping point. Importantly, it should encourage you to read further so that you can easily answer questions from any point of view on that topic.

Consider using this book in the following manner:

- Read the question and then record your answer before you read the correct answer.
- Look at the correct answer and the explanation.
- Read the source reference citation.

Also, read the "High-Yield Facts," a synopsis of significant points presented as condensed summaries. These "High-Yield Facts" highlight key points in pathophysiology for rapid review. They serve also as a "memory jog" when reviewing the questions, and it is important to read the source reference citations accompanying them.

The process of studying remains paramount, not necessarily whether you know the correct answer to one question or many questions. Don't fail to read the source reference citation listed for each question, especially the questions for which you do not readily know the answer. In this manner, you will increase the depth and breadth of your knowledge, which after all is the goal of testing yourself on these questions.

Acknowledgments

Mentors open doors for us in a way that only mentors can do. They promote our career and help us to see its direction. Their interest and understanding make the difference in the paths we take. Several mentors aided me throughout differing times of my career and I want to acknowledge them: Harold Heine, Ph.D., at Bucknell University, my first research mentor; the late Pinckney Jones Harman, Ph.D., at New York University School of Medicine; H. Sherwood Lawrence, M.D., also of New York University School of Medicine, who guided me into a career in infectious disease; Robert M. Chanock, M.D., at the National Institutes of Allergy and Infectious Diseases, who nurtured my research endeavors in virus diseases; Morton D. Bogdonoff, M.D., at the University of Illinois College of Medicine, who encouraged my becoming a Chair of a Department of Medicine; Erling Norrby, M.D., Ph.D., of the Karolinska Institute, Stockholm, Sweden, who opened his laboratory to me for my sabbatical and inspired me; and my wife, Deedee, who guides, encourages, nurtures, and inspires me in all my endeavors, and without whom my career would not have been the joy that it is.

Maurice A. Mufson, M.D., M.A.C.P.
Huntington, West Virginia

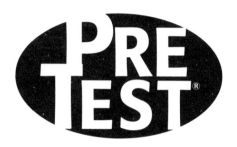

Pathophysiology

PreTest® Self-Assessment and Review

High-Yield Facts in Pathophysiology

1. Many diseases have an immunologic basis. Example: **Graft versus host (GVH) disease** can develop in an immunosuppressed individual who receives immunocompetent donor cells. The donor cells respond to histocompatibility antigens present on the recipient's cells that are NOT found on the donor cells. Bone marrow contains immunocompetent T cells. (*Murray, 5/e, p 123.*)

2. The following chart compares **bacterial meningitis** and **viral meningitis**. (*McPhee, 2/e, pp 61–63.*)

	Bacterial Meningitis	**Viral Meningitis**
Disease state	Acute: significant mortality without antibiotic therapy	Acute: usually self-limited
Symptoms	Fever	Fever
	Worst headache of life	Worst headache of life
	Meningismus	Meningismus
	Mental status changes	Mental status changes
Physical exam findings	Photophobia	Photophobia
	Nausea	Nausea
	Vomiting	Vomiting
	Fever	Fever
	Kernig's sign—positive	Kernig's sign—positive
	Brudinski's sign—positive	Brudinski's sign—positive
Etiology	Neonates	Cocksackie A and B viruses
	Escherichia coli	Poliovirus
	Group B *Streptococcus*	Mumps virus
	Listeria monocytogenes	Epstein-Barr virus
	Children	Adenovirus
	Neisseria meningitidis	Cytomegalovirus
	Streptococcus pneumoniae	
	Haeophilus influenzae, nonimmunized	

	Bacterial Meningitis	**Viral Meningitis**
Etiology (cont'd)	Adults (more than 18 years old) N. meningitidis S. pneumoniae L. monocytogenes Gram-negative bacilli	
Cerebrospinal fluid results	Decreased glucose Increased protein Increased neutrophils Increased pressure	Normal glucose Slightly increased protein Increased monocytes Normal or slightlly increased pressure Gram stain shows no bacteria
Treatment	IV antibiotics Supportive therapy	Supportive therapy
Complications	Cerebral edema Deafness Death	Deafness Weakness

3. Carcinomas undergo phenotypic transition from **normal** → **hyperplasia** → **carcinoma in situ** → **invasive carcinoma** → **metastasis**. Carcinomas occur as a result of a constellation of physiologic and genetic changes (e.g., APC, hMLH1, and hMSH2—colon carcinoma/BRCA1 and BRCA2—breast carcinoma). (*McPhee, 2/e, pp 83–84.*)

4. **Colon carcinoma** begins when cell cycle regulation loses control over growth, and a collection of rapidly multiplying cells (**hyperplasia**) form an adenoma. The adenoma can continue to develop into **carcinoma in situ.** The first evidence of disease may be occult rectal bleeding indicating the appearance of new friable vessels supplying the tumor. Next, the cancer cells invade the basement membrane of the colon (**invasive carcinoma**), gaining access to the body's transport systems (lymphatic and hematogenous). **Metastasis** to lymph nodes and distant body regions can occur. (*McPhee, 2/e, pp 85–87.*)

5. Many malignancies have characteristic indirect systemic effects via multiple mechanisms. In lung malignancies, excess adrenocorticotropic hormone (ACTH) production results in a Cushing-like syn-

drome and excess antidiuretic hormone (ADH) production results in a syndrome of inappropriate antidiuretic hormone secretion (SIADH). Malignancies (e.g., squamous cell carcinoma) can produce peptides related to PTH, causing hypercalcemia. Carcinoid syndromes produce serotonin or prostaglandins that can cause flushing, restrictive lung symptoms, ascites, and hypotension. (*McPhee, 2/e, p 96.*)

6. **Pernicious anemia** occurs when antibodies to intrinsic factor and parietal cells attack the gastric mucosa, causing gastric atrophy. The disruption of the normal function of the gastric mucosa affects vitamin B_{12} absorption on two levels: stomach acid deficiency (achlorhydria) prevents the release of vitamin B_{12} from food digestion, and intrinsic factor is necessary for vitamin B_{12} absorption in the terminal ileum. The chronic loss of vitamin B_{12} results in abnormal RBC maturation without changes in hemoglobin synthesis leading to macrocytic anemia. (*Fauci, 14/e, pp 655–656; McPhee, 2/e, p 111.*)

7. Pathophysiology of hearing loss (*McPhee, 2/e, pp 145–146.*)

Type of Hearing Loss	Etiology	Testing
Conductive deafness	Disruption of conduction and amplification of sound from the external auditory canal to the inner ear	Negative Rinne test Weber test: heard best in the affected ear Audiometry
Sensorineural	Impaired function of inner ear or cranial nerve VIII	Positive Rinne test Weber test: heard best in the unaffected ear Audiometry
Central deafness	Damaged CNS auditory pathways	Audiometry

8. **Myasthenia gravis** is an autoimmune disease characterized by antibodies to acetylcholine receptors, causing a deficiency in the number of acetylcholine receptors on the postsynaptic (muscle) terminal, resulting in reduced efficiency of neuromuscular activity. The disease commonly presents in small muscle groups, accompanied by intermittent fatigue and weakness relieved by rest. (*McPhee, 2/e, pp 152–153.*)

9. **Psoriasis** is an inflammatory parakeratotic accumulation of skin cells that features erythematous, demarcated lesions with scaly patches commonly found on scalp, extensor surfaces of extremities, and fingernails. (*McPhee, 2/e, pp 169–170.*)

10. **Asthma** is an obstructive pulmonary disease characterized by airway narrowing as a result of smooth muscle spasms, inflammation, edema, and thick mucus production. The pathophysiologic response is mediated by local cellular injury, lymphocyte activation (antigen exposure, B cell activation, and cytokine activity), IgE-mediated mast cell (producing histamine, leukotrienes, and platelet-activating factor), and eosinophil activation. (*McPhee, 2/e, pp 200–201.*)

11. Pulmonary function tests: obstructive lung disease vs. restrictive lung disease.

Pulmonary Function Test	Obstructive Lung Diease (e.g., Chronic Obstructive Pulmonary Disease	Restrictive Lung Disease (e.g., Pulmonary Fibrosis
FVC	↓	↓
FEV_1	↓	↓
FEV_1%	↓	Normal / ↑
TLC	↑	↓
RV	↑	Normal / ↓

12. **Pulmonary embolism** occurs when a venous thrombi (usually from a deep vein thrombosis) lodges in the pulmonary circulation. The pathophysiology includes hemodynamic changes, increased alveolar dead space with increased ventilation/perfusion ratios, and decreased oxygen perfusion to body tissues. Common acute presentations include tachypnea, hemoptysis, tachycardia, fever, cough, and pleuritic pain. (*McPhee, 2/e, pp 214–216.*)

13. In normal individuals, as left ventricular end-diastolic pressure or preload increases, stroke volume will increase proportionately. In patients who suffer heart failure, increased left ventricular end-diastolic pressure is not met with increased stroke volume, because the contractility is depressed and is unable to function; thus, the patient ultimately experiences heart failure. Frank-Starling curves or ventricular function

curves are diagrams that show the relationship between stroke volume or cardiac output and preload or left ventricular end-diastolic volume. (*Lilly, p 150.*)

14. **Stable angina** is caused by a fixed partial atherosclerotic plaque in one or more of coronary arteries. When at rest, blood flow is able to provide adequate oxygenation to the heart muscle. On exertion, oxygen demand increases. The partial occlusion prevents adequate oxygenation to the heart, resulting in chest discomfort. Unstable angina is caused by thrombus formation on a fissuring atherosclerotic plaque, which transiently prevents adequate oxygenation to the heart. The resulting ischemia causes chest discomfort whether at rest or during exertion. (*McPhee, 2/e, pp 246–248.*)

15. Chronic esophageal reflux (as a result of a transient weakened lower esophageal sphincter, alcohol use, and tobacco abuse) can result in **Barrett's esophagus.** In the disease, columnar epithelium replaces normal squamous epithelium. Individuals with Barrett's esophagus have an increased risk of developing adenocarcinoma of the esophagus. (*McPhee, 2/e, p 306.*)

16. **Helicobacter pylori** is a common bacteria that infects the gastric mucosa, providing an increased propensity for peptic ulcer disease through inflammatory mechanisms. Other risk factors for peptic ulcer disease are use of a nonsteroidal anti-inflammatory drug (NSAID), family history, smoking, and Zollinger-Ellison syndrome (gastrinoma). (*McPhee, 2/e, p 307.*)

17. **Crohn's disease** is a chronic inflammatory bowel disease that affects the whole gastrointestinal tract (from mouth to anus) and is distinguished by **alternating regions** ("skip lesions") of normal bowel and full-thickness ulcerations and granuloma formation of the bowel wall. Common manifestations are bloody diarrhea, fistula, iritis, arthritis, abscess formation, and small bowel obstruction. (*McPhee, 2/e, p 315.*)

18. **Ulcerative colitis** is an inflammatory bowel disease that causes **continuous,** partial-thickness (mucosa only) ulcerations of all or part of the colon and is manifested by bloody diarrhea and abdominal pain. (*McPhee, 2/e, pp 315–316.*)

19. **Type 1 diabetes mellitus** (previously called insulin-dependent diabetes mellitus) and **type 2 diabetes mellitus** (previously called non-insulin-

dependent diabetes) differ in multiple ways. Type 1 DM usually starts in young (less than 30 years old), nonobese individuals who sometimes have a family history (weak genetic component). Insulin production deficiency predominates, with rare insulin receptor resistance. Type 1 DM is always treated with exogenous insulin. Diabetic ketoacidosis is a common complication. Type 2 DM usually starts in older (more than 40 years old), obese individuals who often have a family history of disease (strong genetic component). Recently, type 2 DM has been seen in younger adults and children, probably due to a change in life style. Insulin resistance is a major feature. Type 2 DM is often treated with exogenous insulin. Hyperosmolar coma is a common complication. (*McPhee, 2/e, pp 431–445.*)

20. **Hyperthyroidism** is characterized by sweating, agitation, weight loss, heat intolerance, palpitations, irritability, and dyspnea. Triiodothyronine (T_3) and thyroxine (T_4) are elevated with concurrent depression of thyroid-stimulating hormone (TSH). Hypothyroidism is characterized by fatigue, depression, constipation, weight gain, decreased sweating, cold intolerance, and hoarseness. T_3 and T_4 are depressed with concurrent elevation of TSH. (*McPhee, 2/e, pp 475–483.*)

21. **Cushing's syndrome** (excessive cortisol production) is characterized by moon facies, neck/trunk obesity, weight gain, mental status changes, purple striae on abdomen, osteoporosis, and glucose intolerance. Often there is excess ACTH production from the pituitary (Cushing's disease) or from tumors (ectopic ACTH). (*McPhee, 2/e, p 497.*)

22. **Conn's syndrome** (excessive mineralocorticoid secretion) is characterized by hypokalemia, hypertension, metabolic alkalosis, glucose intolerance, and weakness. (*McPhee, 2/e, p 497.*)

23. **Addison's disease** (primary adrenal insufficiency) is characterized by weakness, fatigue, weight loss, hypotension, cold intolerance, abdominal pain, diarrhea, anorexia, hyperkalemia, hyponatremia, and hypoglycemia. (*McPhee, 2/e, p 497.*)

24. **Preeclampsia-eclampsia** is characterized by hypertension, proteinuria, and edema after week 20 of pregnancy. Without treatment, a pattern of complications occurs. Complications include bleeding, malignant hypertension, stroke, renal failure, seizures, disseminated intravascular coagulation, and death. (*McPhee, 2/e, pp 539–540.*)

25. **Minimal change disease** is the most common cause of nephrotic syndrome in children and is characterized by isolated proteinuria (more than 3.5 g of protein in 24-h urine) and obliterated epithelial podocytes on the glomerular basement membrane. *(Fauci, 14/e, pp 1540–1541.)*

26. **Human immunodeficiency infection (HIV) and acquired immunodeficiency disease (AIDS).** HIV infection occurs worldwide. It is mainly a sexually transmitted disease that can be transmitted by blood and blood products contaminated with the virus. The diagnosis of AIDS is made when any AIDS defining illness occurs in a person with HIV, such as **Pneumocystis carinii pneumonia (PCP)**, thrush due to *Candida,* or their CD4 lymphocyte count drops below 200 cells/μL. AIDS is the leading cause of death in persons 25–44 years old in the United States. HIV infection begins with an acute HIV syndrome, latency ensues, and then early symptomatic illness and eventually fully symptomatic illness with a myriad of complicating infections and noninfectious diseases. The entire cycle occurs over a period of more than 10–15 years, and possibly longer now that effective treatment regimens are available. The treatment of HIV and AIDS can alter this progression and provide long periods free of detectable viral loads, almost normal CD4 lymphocyte counts and good quality of life. Treatment changes rapidly on the basis of the introduction of new anti-HIV drugs and new protocols specifying their use. The standard of care now is three-drug regimens (triple therapy). *(Fauci, 14/e, pp 1791–1825.)*

Immune System

Questions

DIRECTIONS: Each item below contains a question or incomplete statement followed by suggested responses. Select the **one best** response to each question.

1. The major immunoglobulin class in normal adult human serum is

a. IgA
b. IgG
c. IgM
d. IgE
e. IgD

2. The predominant antibody found in a primary immune response is

a. IgA
b. IgG
c. IgM
d. IgE
e. IgD

3. Which immunoglobulin class is found on the surface of mast cells?

a. IgA
b. IgG
c. IgM
d. IgE
e. IgD

4. Which immunoglobulin class is a major component of mucosal secretions?

a. IgA
b. IgG
c. IgM
d. IgE
e. IgD

5. Which immunoglobulin class can cross the placenta?

a. IgA
b. IgG
c. IgM
d. IgE
e. IgD

6. Which of the following cells are important in an innate immune response to extracellular bacteria?

a. T lymphocytes
b. B lymphocytes
c. Neutrophils
d. Eosinophils
e. Mast cells

7. Which one of the following is the most potent and effective antigen-presenting cell (APC)?

a. Monocytes-macrophages
b. Mast cells
c. T lymphocytes
d. B lymphocytes
e. Dendritic-Langerhans cells

8. Compared with a healthy individual, lymph nodes from a person with a deficiency in B lymphocytes would have

a. Few or no primary follicles
b. Enlarged germinal centers
c. Few Howell-Jolly bodies
d. No paracortex
e. Increased number of Heinz bodies

9. A newborn infected with group B streptococcus would produce and secrete antibody of which of the following class(es)?

a. IgM only
b. IgG only
c. IgM and IgG
d. Neither IgM nor IgG
e. IgA only

10. Eosinophils are associated with the defense against infections caused by

a. Virus
b. Intracellular bacteria
c. Extracellular bacteria
d. Invasive parasites
e. Mycoplasma

11. To determine whether a fetus acquired an infection in utero, antigen-specific antibody to which of the following classes should be measured?

a. IgA
b. IgM
c. IgG
d. IgD
e. IgE

12. During an immune response, antibodies are made against different structures (usually proteins) on an infectious agent. These structures are referred to as

a. Adjuvants
b. Allotypes
c. Isotypes
d. Epitopes
e. Alleles

13. Which one of the following complement components enhances phagocytosis of bacteria by opsonization?

a. C1
b. Factor B
c. C3b
d. C5a
e. C5b6789

14. Which one of the following complement components mediates cytolysis?

a. C1
b. Factor B
c. C3b
d. C5a
e. C5b6789

15. Which one of the following complement components is a chemo-attractant for neutrophils?

a. C1
b. Factor B
c. C3b
d. C5a
e. C5b6789

16. Which one of the following complement components binds to anti-body to activate the classical pathway?

a. C1
b. Factor B
c. C3b
d. C5a
e. C5b6789

17. A patient with a predisposition for disseminated infections by *Neisseria* bacteria may have a deficiency in

a. Membrane attack complex formation (C5 to C9)
b. Classical pathway activation
c. C3
d. C1 inhibitor
e. C4

18. Which one of the following complement component deficiencies is associated with individuals with frequent pyogenic bacterial infections?

a. Membrane attack complex (C5 to C9)
b. C1 inhibitor
c. C2
d. C3
e. C4

19. A person with an abnormality in which one of the following early complement components would most likely experience the most serious clinical manifestations?

a. C1
b. C2
c. C3
d. Factor B
e. C1 inhibitor

20. A 6-year-old boy has received a deep puncture wound while playing in his neighbor's yard. His records indicate that he has had the standard DPT immunizations and a booster when he entered school. What is the most appropriate therapy for this child?

a. Tetanus toxoid
b. Tetanus antitoxin
c. Both toxoid and antitoxin at the same site
d. Toxoid and antitoxin at different sites
e. No treatment

21. Toxic shock syndrome toxin-1 is produced by some strains of *S. aureus* and is thought to be responsible for the clinical manifestations of disease by this organism. This toxin is referred to as a superantigen because it can

a. Activate T cells in an antigen-nonspecific manner
b. Activate B cells without T cell help
c. Become immunogenic when attached to a carrier protein
d. Prolong the presence of antigen in a tissue
e. Evoke IgE

22. Neutralizing antiviral antibody produced in response to infection by an enveloped virus acts on which one of the following components of the virus?

a. Matrix proteins
b. One or more surface glycoproteins
c. Internal protein components
d. Nucleic acid
e. Internal nonprotein components

23. Direct killing of cells infected with virus is usually accomplished by

a. CD8-positive T cells
b. CD4-positive T helper 1 cells
c. CD4-positive T helper 2 cells
d. plasma cells
e. CD19-positive B cells

24. *Mycobacterium tuberculosis* results in an intracellular bacterial infection that provokes which one of the following immune responses?
a. Natural killer cytotoxic response
b. CD8-positive cytotoxic T cell response
c. T helper 1 delayed type hypersensitivity response
d. Complement mediated lysis of infected cell
e. Eosinophilia

25. Which one of the following is a B cell neoplasm?
a. Non-Hodgkin's lymphoma
b. Acute lymphoblastic leukemia
c. Burkitt's lymphoma
d. Hodgkin's disease
e. Histiocytosis X

26. During an immune response to pathogens in the intestine, the primary function of M cells along the Peyer's patches is to
a. Transport antigen to lymphocytes
b. Produce antigen-specific IgA antibody
c. Present antigen to lymphocytes
d. Secrete cytokines to "help" in antibody production
e. Secrete chemokines

27. Which one of the following tests is used for the determination of the titer of antihepatitis B antibody?
a. Flow cytometry (FACS)
b. Enzyme-linked immunosorbent assay (ELISA)
c. Latex agglutination
d. Coombs' test
e. Mixed lymphocyte reaction

28. Which one of the following tests is used for the detection of anti-Rh antibody in blood?
a. Flow cytometry (FACS)
b. Enzyme-linked immunosorbent assay (ELISA)
c. Latex agglutination
d. Coombs' test
e. Mixed lymphocyte reaction

29. Which one of the following tests is used for the assessment of the level of CD4+ T lymphocytes in an HIV-infected patient?

a. Flow cytometry (FACS)
b. Enzyme-linked immunosorbent assay (ELISA)
c. Latex agglutination
d. Coombs' test
e. Mixed lymphocyte reaction

30. Which one of the following tests is used for the evaluating the degree of compatibility between donor and patient lymphocytes?

a. Flow cytometry (FACS)
b. Enzyme-linked immunosorbent assay (ELISA)
c. Latex agglutination
d. Coombs' test
e. Mixed lymphocyte reaction

31. Which one of the following tests is used for the detection of group A streptococci from a throat swab?

a. Flow cytometry (FACS)
b. Enzyme-linked immunosorbent assay (ELISA)
c. Latex agglutination
d. Coombs' test
e. Mixed lymphocyte reaction

32. Which hypersensitivity reaction is associated with Goodpasture's syndrome?

a. Type I: immediate
b. Type II: cytotoxic
c. Type III: immune complex
d. Type IV: cell mediated

33. Which hypersensitivity reaction is associated with serum sickness?

a. Type I: immediate
b. Type II: cytotoxic
c. Type III: immune complex
d. Type IV: cell mediated

34. Which hypersensitivity reaction is associated with a tuberculin reaction?

a. Type I: immediate
b. Type II: cytotoxic
c. Type III: immune complex
d. Type IV: cell mediated

35. Which hypersensitivity reaction is associated with poison ivy?

a. Type I: immediate
b. Type II: cytotoxic
c. Type III: immune complex
d. Type IV: cell mediated

36. Which hypersensitivity reaction is associated with an anaphylactic reaction after a bee sting?

a. Type I: immediate
b. Type II: cytotoxic
c. Type III: immune complex
d. Type IV: cell mediated

37. Which hypersensitivity reaction is associated with hemolytic disease of the newborn?

a. Type I: immediate
b. Type II: cytotoxic
c. Type III: immune complex
d. Type IV: cell mediated

38. Which hypersensitivity reaction is associated with poststreptococcal glomerulonephritis?

a. Type I: immediate
b. Type II: cytotoxic
c. Type III: immune complex
d. Type IV: cell mediated

39. A patient with recurrent infections with yeast and the incapacity to control viral infections may indicate a deficiency in

a. Cellular immunity
b. Complement
c. Granulocytes
d. Humoral immunity
e. Eosinophils

40. Graft versus host disease can be a complication of which of the following kinds of transplantation?

a. Kidney
b. Bone marrow
c. Liver
d. Skin
e. Cornea

41. Which cytokine promotes the proliferation of T and B lymphocytes?

a. IFN-γ (interferon γ)
b. IL-2 (interleukin 2)
c. IL-4 (interleukin 4)
d. TNF-α (tumor necrosis factor α)
e. TGF-β (transforming growth factor β)

42. Which cytokine promotes various biologic actions associated with inflammation?

a. IFN-γ (interferon γ)
b. IL-2 (interleukin 2)
c. IL-4 (interleukin 4)
d. TNF-α (tumor necrosis factor α)
e. TGF-β (transforming growth factor β)

43. Which cytokine antagonizes or suppresses many responses of lymphocytes?

a. IFN-γ (interferon γ)
b. IL-2 (interleukin 2)
c. IL-4 (interleukin 4)
d. TNF-α (tumor necrosis factor α)
e. TGF-β (transforming growth factor β)

44. Which cytokine functions as a promotor of T helper 2 (T_H2) development and IgE synthesis?

a. IFN-γ (interferon γ)
b. IL-2 (interleukin 2)
c. IL-4 (interleukin 4)
d. TNF-α (tumor necrosis factor α)
e. TGF-β (transforming growth factor β)

45. Which cytokine functions as an activator of macrophages and natural killer (NK) cells?

a. IFN-γ (interferon γ)
b. IL-2 (interleukin 2)
c. IL-4 (interleukin 4)
d. TNF-α (tumor necrosis factor α)
e. TGF-β (transforming growth factor β)

Immune System

Answers

1. The answer is b. (*Murray, 5/e, p 93.*) IgG makes up about 85% of the immunoglobulin in adult serum.

2. The answer is c. (*Murray, 5/e, p 93.*) Most of the antibody produced in a primary immune response is IgM. As time passes or at a second encounter with the same antigen, isotype (class) switching can occur.

3. The answer is d. (*Murray, 5/e, p 93.*) IgE is found on the surface of mast cells and basophils. When antigen binds to the IgE, the mast cell releases various mediators involved in allergic reactions and antiparasitic defense.

4. The answer is a. (*Murray, 5/e, p 93.*) IgA is the predominant immunoglobulin class in mucosal secretions such as saliva, colostrum, bronchial, and genitourinary tract secretions. It is often called secretory immunoglobulin.

5. The answer is b. (*Murray, 5/e, p 93.*) IgG can cross the placenta and confer passive immunity to the fetus and newborn.

6. The answer is c. (*Murray, 5/e, p 110–111.*) Innate immunity involves antigen-nonspecific immune defense. Neutrophils circulate in the blood and can migrate into tissue to ingest and kill bacteria. Although T and B cells can augment the innate immune response, they become inactivated in an antigen-specific manner. Eosinophils, also part of the innate immune response, are important in parasitic, rather than bacterial, infections.

7. The answer is e. (*Fauci, 14/e, p 1767.*) Dendritic/Langerhans cells are the most potent and effective antigen-presenting cells (APC). The other cells do not possess as effective an antigen-presenting capability.

8. The answer is a. (*Murray, 5/e, p 86.*) The major cell type within follicles is the B cell; a germinal center is a follicle where cells are undergoing active proliferation. A deficiency in B cells would result in decreased size and number of follicles. The paracortex is predominately a T cell area. Heinz bodies (red cell inclusion body of denatured hemoglobin) and Howell-Jolly bodies (red cell inclusion body of parasites) are found in the spleen.

9. The answer is a. *(Roitt, 5/e, p 168.)* A normal newborn can make IgM antibody in response to challenge with antigen. If IgG is detected in the newborn, it is most likely the result of placental transfer from the mother.

10. The answer is d. *(Fauci, 14/e, p 358.)* Eosinophils are associated with invasive parasitic infections. They localize near the parasite, degranulate, and release antiparasitic molecules. Eosinophils do not exhibit any effective function against intracellular bacteria or virus, which reside within host cells, or mycoplasma. Neutrophils are usually associated with extracellular bacterial infections.

11. The answer is b. *(Roitt, 5/e, p 168.)* The fetus and newborn infant can only produce measurable IgM antibody in response to infection. If IgG is detected, it is the result of an immune response by the mother and the antibody has crossed the placenta.

12. The answer is d. *(Murray, 5/e, p 88, 121.)* Usually an immunogen contains more than one molecule that can elicit an antibody response. These different molecules are called epitopes (or antigenic determinants) and are the structures with which antibodies react. Isotypes refer to the different classes of immunoglobulins (e.g., IgM, IgG, and IgA). Allotypes refer to isotypes that differ among individuals within a species. Adjuvants are substances that can enhance an immune response to antigen. Alleles are variations of a gene.

13. The answer is c. *(Murray, 5/e, pp 98–99.)* The cleavage component of C3, C3b, when bound to the surface of a cell, promotes the phagocytosis of that cell by a process referred to as opsonization.

14. The answer is e. *(Murray, 5/e, pp 98–99.)* Complement components C5b, 6, 7, 8, and 9 associate to generate the membrane attack complex (MAC) that disrupts the integrity of the cell membrane on which it is formed.

15. The answer is d. (*Murray, 5/e, pp 98–99.*) Several complement cleavage products promote inflammatory responses: C3a, C4a, and C5a. They can also induce the degranulation of mast cells and so are also referred to as anaphylatoxins. C5a has the additional property whereby it is a neutrophil-chemoattracting substance.

16. The answer is a. (*Murray, 5/e, pp 98–99.*) The classical pathway is initiated by antigen-antibody complexes. Binding of C1 to the complex activates the complement cascade.

17. The answer is a. (*Fauci, 14/e, pp 911–912.*) Patients with a familial deficiency in the terminal complement components fail to assemble the membrane attack complex (C5–C9), and they are at risk for disseminated *Neisseria* infections, including attacks of recurrent meningococcal disease. The other components of the complement system do not play a role in this unique susceptibility.

18. The answer is d. (*Fauci, 14/e, p 1771.*) Individuals with C3 deficiency have recurrent serious pyogenic bacterial infections that can be fatal. The absence of C3 leads to the inability to generate the opsonin, C3b, which, when deposited on the surface of the bacteria, promotes phagocytosis. Membrane attack complex deficiencies can lead to disseminated *Neisseria* infections. A deficiency in C1 inhibitor is associated with hereditary angioneurotic edema (HANE). Individuals with C2 deficiency have a predisposition for immune complex disease such as systemic lupus erythematosus.

19. The answer is c. (*Murray, 5/e, p 98.*) C3 plays a central role in both the classical and alternate pathways. An abnormality in this component would disrupt both pathways. C1 and C2 are used only by the classical pathway; therefore, an abnormality in either one or both of these components would leave the alternate pathway intact. Likewise, a defect in factor B (a component of the alternate pathway) would still permit the activation of the classical pathway.

20. The answer is e. (*Murray, 5/e, pp 128–129.*) Because the boy received his booster within the last 2 years, his level of immunity should be adequate. If an individual has no history of immunization, both antitoxin (passive immunization with tetanus immune globulin) for temporary and fast protection and toxoid (toxin detoxified with formaldehyde) for future and long-lasting protection should be given at different sites.

21. The answer is a. *(Fauci, 14/e, p 877.)* A superantigen can activate T cells without binding to the T cell receptor in an antigen-specific manner. Therefore, the superantigen can stimulate a large number of T cells, which can result in massive cytokine release, causing shock and tissue damage. An antigen that can activate B cells without T cell help is called a T-independent antigen. Haptens, usually small molecules, can become antigenic when attached to carrier proteins. Adjuvants can help in maintaining antigen at a tissue site. It does not evoke IgE, which is found in allergic reactions.

22. The answer is b. *(Fauci, 14/e, p 1070.)* During infection by enveloped viruses, antibody is produced, which reacts with the surface glycoproteins to neutralize the virus. Neutralizing antibody does not react with the other components of the virus. Usually, neutralizing (or protective) antibody is formed to surface components of the virus and not internal components.

23. The answer is a. *(Murray, 5/e, p 119.)* CD8-positive T cells are cytolytic T cells that can respond to viral peptides/MHC class I complexes on infected cells. CD4-positive T helper 1 cells usually function by releasing cytokines that promote an inflammatory response. CD4-positive T helper 2 cells produce cytokines important in generating antibody production. Plasma cells secrete antibody. CD19-positive B cells regulate B cell activation.

24. The answer is c. *(Murray, 5/e, p 114.)* Delayed type hypersensitivity (DTH) responses are important in protection against intracellular bacteria. In this type of response, macrophages and other inflammatory processes are activated to kill the infected cell. NK cells, cytotoxic T cells, and complement do not seem to provide adequate protection against intracellular bacteria. Eosinophilia occurs in allergy reactions.

25. The answer is c. *(Fauci, 2/e, pp 1090–1091, 1754–1755.)* Burkitt's lymphoma is a B cell neoplasm associated with Epstein-Barr virus (EBV) infection in about 15% of the disease in the United States and about 90%

of the disease in Africa. Hodgkin's disease and histiocytosis X are monocyte neoplasms, and non-Hodgkin's lymphoma and acute lymphoblastic leukemia are T cell neoplasms.

26. The answer is a. (*Murray, 5/e, p 87.*) M cells deliver antigen to Peyer's patches, but they do not act as antigen-presenting cells to lymphocytes. Antibody is made by B cells within the Peyer's patch. T helper 2 cells are the main source of cytokines functioning in helping B cells make and secrete antibody.

27. The answer is b. (*Murray, 5/e, pp 147, 149.*) ELISA can be used to determine the relative antibody concentration to a specific antigen (titer); the assay can also be used to quantitate antibody.

28. The answer is d. (*Roitt, 5/e, pp 322–324.*) An indirect Coombs' test is used to detect circulating anti-Rh antibody: anti-Rh antibody reacts with Rh+ erythrocytes causing agglutination of the erythrocytes. The direct Coombs' tests for cell-bound anti-Rh antibody.

29. The answer is a. (*Murray, 5/e, pp 146, 147.*) In flow cytometry, cells in suspension tagged with fluorescent-labeled antibody can be identified and quantitated.

30. The answer is e. (*Roitt, 5/e, pp 361–362.*) A mixed lymphocyte reaction assays the histocompatibility between two individuals. Donor cells are treated to prevent DNA synthesis and proliferation. The recipient's cells are mixed with the donor's cells. If the donor's cells express foreign MHC antigens, the recipient's lymphocytes will proliferate. Proliferation can be measured by the uptake of radioactive thymidine.

31. The answer is c. (*Murray, 5/e, pp 145, 195.*) In a latex agglutination test, antigen-specific antibody is attached to latex beads. When the beads are mixed with a specimen containing antigen, the beads agglutinate, which can be detected visually.

32. The answer is b. (*Murray, 5/e, pp 123–124.*) The hypersensitivity reaction in Goodpasture's syndrome is type II in which antibody mediates cell lysis. Antiglomerular basement membrane antibody is cytotoxic. In

Goodpasture's syndrome, antibody forms to lung and kidney basement membranes causing damage to the tissue.

33. The answer is c. (*Murray, 5/e, pp 123–125.*) Serum sickness results from the injection of serum made in non-human species into humans. Antibody to the soluble nonhuman proteins are generated and immune complexes form. The complexes are trapped in capillaries and initiate an inflammatory response that causes damage to tissue.

34. The answer is d. (*Murray, 5/e, p 125.*) Antigen injected intradermally into a previously sensitized individual elicits a delayed type hypersensitivity response. This involves the recruitment of CD4+ T lymphocytes and macrophages to the site.

35. The answer is d. (*Murray, 5/e, p 125.*) Poison ivy, an allergic contact dermatitis, is a delayed hypersensitivity reaction mediated by CD4+ T lymphocytes in the skin.

36. The answer is a. (*Murray, 5/e, p 123.*) Anaphylaxis is a severe immediate hypersensitivity response. IgE, produced at the time of initial exposure to antigen (bee venom), binds to mast cells. On subsequent exposure, the antigen (bee venom) reacts with the mast cell-bound IgE, leading to the release of mediators from the mast cells. The mediators produce the symptoms associated with the anaphylactic reaction.

37. The answer is b. (*Murray, 5/e, pp 123–124.*) This is a cytotoxic hypersensitivity reaction in which IgG anti-Rh antibody, produced in a previous pregnancy, crosses the placenta and binds to Rh+ fetal red blood cells. This triggers the classical complement pathway leading to the lysis of the fetal red cells.

38. The answer is c. (*Murray, 5/e, pp 123–124, 195.*) Complexes of bacterial antigen and antibody form and become trapped in the renal vasculature. Complement is activated and neutrophils are recruited to the site. During the process of removal of the immune complexes, tissue damage may occur.

39. The answer is a. (*Murray, 5/e, pp 126–127.*) Individuals with T cell deficiencies are susceptible to infections with microbes that reside within host cells (virus, *Mycobacterium* species, and fungi). Humoral immune deficiency or complement deficiency usually results in recurrent bacterial, rather than viral, infections. Granulocyte deficiency may also result in bacterial and yeast infections. Because the statement indicates that the patient has problems with viral infections, the best answer is a deficiency in T cell immunity.

40. The answer is b. *(Murray, 5/e, p 123.)* Graft versus host (GVH) disease can develop in an immunosuppressed individual who receives immunocompetent donor cells. The donor cells respond to histocompatibility antigens present on the recipient's cells, which are NOT found on the donor cells. Bone marrow contains immunocompetent T cells; liver, kidney, and skin do not have a sufficient number of immunocompetent T cells to elicit GVH reactions. Corneal transplants do not evoke GVH.

41. The answer is b. *(Murray, 5/e, p 81.)* IL-2 acts on T cells to induce their progression through the cell cycle; it also acts as a growth factor for B cells.

42. The answer is d. *(Murray, 5/e, p 81.)* TNF-α activities depend partly on the quantity of cytokine produced. TNF-α is also associated with the production of IL-1 and IL-6. At low levels, it induces a local inflammatory effect by stimulating leukocyte recruitment. At moderate levels, it can have systemic effects, inducing fever and acute-phase protein synthesis within the liver. At high quantities, TNF-α (in conjunction with IL-1 and IL-6) can produce septic shock syndrome.

43. The answer is e. *(Murray, 5/e, p 81.)* TGF-β seems to be a signal that "turns off" inflammatory or immune responses.

44. The answer is c. *(Murray, 5/e, p 81.)* IL-4 promotes the development of the T helper 2 subset of CD4+ T lymphocytes. It also is important for class switching to IgE.

45. The answer is a. *(Murray, 5/e, p 81.)* IFN-γ acts on macrophages to enhance killing of ingested microbes. It also stimulates the cytolytic activity of NK cells.

Genetic Disease

Questions

DIRECTIONS: Each item contains a question or incomplete statement followed by suggested responses. Select the **one best** response to each question.

46. A patient who has the autosomal dominant gene for type I osteogenesis imperfecta has blue scleras and slightly reduced height, whereas his brother has multiple fractures and deformities. This is an example of

a. Polymorphism
b. Mutation
c. Variable expressivity
d. Fitness

47. Your patient has an autosomal dominantly inherited disease. The patient and his grandfather show evidence of disease, but the patient's father is asymptomatic. This is an example of

a. Polymorphism
b. Mutation
c. Variable expressivity
d. Reduced penetrance

48. Two patients have the same eye color. They have the same

a. HLA type
b. Phenotype
c. Haplotype
d. Mutation

49. A patient has an X-linked disease. His three sisters do not have the disease. He most likely has

a. A mutant recessive gene on the X chromosome
b. A mutant dominant gene on the X chromosome
c. A mutant recessive gene on the Y chromosome
d. A mutant dominant gene on the Y chromosome

50. The fact that type IV osteogenesis imperfecta can be caused by defects on *COLIA* 1 and *COLIA* 2 is an example of

a. Gonadal mosaicism
b. Genetic heterogeneity
c. Allelic heterogeneity
d. Polymorphism

51. In genetics, fitness refers to

a. Strong healthy chromosomes
b. Genes fitting together on a single chromosome
c. Absence of mutations
d. Likelihood of reproduction by the individual with the mutant allele

52. The increased frequency of the recessive gene for sickle cell anemia in the African population is an example of

a. Hypomorphism
b. Hypermorphism
c. Heterozygote advantage
d. Phenotypic heterogeneity

53. Mutations that cause a gain in function of the mutated allele are

a. Hypermorphic
b. Neomorphic
c. Amorphic
d. Hypomorphic

54. When two copies of a mutant allele produce a phenotype more severe than one mutant and one normal copy, we have

a. Dominant inheritance
b. Recessive inheritance
c. Semidominant inheritance
d. Double dominant inheritance

55. Cystic fibrosis

a. Occurs mainly in African Americans
b. Causes endocrine problems with the pancreas gland
c. Is an autosomal recessive disorder
d. Is caused by loss of function mutations in a sodium channel

56. Your patient presents with multiple café au lait spots and neurofibromas. His father and mother do not have neurofibromas. This may be an example of

a. A new mutation
b. Hypermorphism
c. A dominant negative mutation
d. Antimorphism

57. A patient has muscular weakness. His parents and sister do not have weakness, but his mother's brother has weakness. You suspect Duchenne's muscular dystrophy. This is an example of

a. Autosomal recessive inheritance
b. X-linked recessive inheritance
c. Semidominant inheritance
d. Autosomal dominant inheritance

58. Which of the following conditions is known to be multifactorial in etiology and not due to a single gene disorder?

a. Neurofibromatosis
b. Osteogenesis imperfecta
c. Atherosclerosis
d. Cystic fibrosis

59. A 13-year-old child with blue scleras, mildly short stature, and no deformity with a history significant for 10 fractured bones most likely has

a. Type I osteogenesis imperfecta
b. Type II osteogenesis imperfecta
c. Type III osteogenesis imperfecta
d. Type IV osteogenesis imperfecta

60. An infant with multiple fractures, bony deformity, blue scleras, wormian bones in the skull, and beaded ribs died of respiratory difficulties. He most likely had

a. Type I osteogenesis imperfecta
b. Type II osteogenesis imperfecta
c. Type III osteogenesis imperfecta
d. Type IV osteogenesis imperfecta

61. Fragile X-associated mental retardation syndrome

a. Is transmitted from father to son
b. Affects females and males equally
c. 20% of carrier males show no sign of the syndrome
d. Involves a nonrepetitive segment of DNA

62. Which is true regarding CpG islands?

a. They are less than 100 base pairs in length
b. They contain few sites for DNA methylation
c. The island at Xq27.3 is normally unmethylated in male cells but methylated in one of the two X chromosomes in female cells
d. Unmethylation of the CpG island in males correlates with expression of the fragile X-associated mental retardation syndrome

63. A patient has fragile X-associated mental retardation syndrome phenotype. Diagnostic testing of 10^7 lymphocytes reveals repetition of $(5'CGG-3')_n$ segment of DNA where $n > 200$, but variable in number. This variation in number is described as

a. Genetic mosaicism
b. Genetic anticipation
c. Fitness
d. Dosage compensation

64. The FMR1 protein

a. Is expressed in fragile X-associated mental retardation
b. Is normally found in brain and ovaries
c. When defective, is not sufficient to cause the fragile X-associated mental retardation syndrome
d. Is coded by the *FMR1* gene which has the $(5'-CGG-3')_n$ repeat segments

65. A premutation allele

a. If transmitted by a female expands to a full mutation with a likelihood proportionate to the size of the repeat segment
b. If transmitted by a male usually expands to a full mutation regardless of the length of the repeat sequence
c. Causes a change in phenotype
d. Is present in the "carrier" males

66. Fragile X, spinocerebellar ataxia 1, spinobulbar muscular atrophy, and Huntington's chorea

a. All involve synthesis of an altered protein with an expanded polyglutamine region
b. All involve failure to synthesize a protein
c. All involve amplification of an unstable triplet repeat
d. Involve mutation of the *FMR1* gene

67. In the case of a dominant allele

a. Two copies of the allele are needed to produce the altered phenotype
b. One copy of the allele is sufficient to produce the phenotype
c. An offspring with one parent having a dominant allele has a 25% chance of inheriting the dominant allele
d. If two parents have a dominant allele, the offspring has a 50% chance of inheriting the dominant allele

68. The human genome is estimated to contain about how many genes?

a. 25,000
b. 50,000 to 100,000
c. 200,000
d. 225,000

69. Which one of the following genetic diseases is a chromosomal disorder?

a. Cystic fibrosis
b. Hemochromatosis
c. Klinefelter's syndrome
d. Hemophilia
e. Fragile-X

70. Most children with Down's syndrome are

a. Born to women under 35
b. Born to women over 35
c. Tall
d. Underweight

71. In Down's syndrome, life expectancy is characterized as

a. 90% survive to age 30 regardless of the presence of congenital heart disease
b. 60% survive to age 10 and 50% survive to age 30 if congenital heart disease is present
c. It is the same as unaffected individuals if congenital heart disease is absent
d. 90% die of Alzheimer's disease by age 20

72. Which is true of Down's syndrome?

a. 50% of cases are caused by an extra maternal chromosome
b. 25% of nondysjunction occur in meiosis I
c. Maternal and paternal nondysjunction events are associated with advanced maternal age
d. It is impossible to tell whether the extra gene came from the mother or the father

73. The dietary treatment of phenylketonuria must be initiated when?

a. Before the child is 3 weeks of age
b. The child is 4 to 6 weeks of age
c. The child is 7 to 10 weeks of age
d. Between 3 and 6 months of age

74. Newborn screening for phenylketonuria

a. Occurs at 7 days after birth
b. Confirms the diagnosis in about 5% of those screened
c. Has a false-negative rate of 1:70
d. Shows a prevalence in the general population of 1:50,000

75. Which treatment regimen is appropriate for phenylketonuria?

a. Infants are fed a semisynthetic formula low in phenylalanine
b. Breast feeding is prohibited
c. Infants are fed a diet totally devoid of phenylalanine
d. It can be discontinued at age 18

76. The neurologic deficits of phenylketonuria are due to

a. Primarily the metabolites of phenylalanine
b. A direct effect of phenylalanine on energy production, protein synthesis, and neurotransmitter homeostasis
c. Phenylalanine causing an increased transport of neutral amino acids across the blood-brain barrier
d. The increased action of phenylalanine hydroxylase

77. In phenylketonuria, phenylalanine is a competitive inhibitor of which enzyme that, when blocked, contributes to the hypopigmentation of hair and skin?

a. Cystathionase
b. Tyrosinase
c. 4-Hydroxyphenylpyruvate dioxygenase
d. Sarcosine dehydrogenase
e. Histidine ammonia lyase

78. The different genetic forms of phenylketonuria illustrate two different pathophysiologic mechanisms by which inborn errors of metabolism cause disease. These are

a. End-product overproduction and substrate accumulation
b. End-product deficiency and substrate accumulation
c. End-product overproduction and substrate deficiency
d. End-product deficiency and substrate deficiency

79. Regarding the centimorgan

a. The human genome is composed of approximately 6000 centimorgans in recombination distance
b. It is a measure of genetic distance that reflects the probability of a crossover between two loci during meiosis
c. One centimorgan approximates a 5% chance of a crossover during meiosis
d. The average chromosome contains about 500 centimorgans of genetic material

80. The likelihood of two parents producing two offspring with identical chromosomes (other than by twinning) is

a. 1:540,000
b. 1:1,200,000
c. 1:5,800,000
d. 1:8,400,000

81. A mutation in which the base replacement changes the codon for one amino acid to another is called a

a. Missense mutation
b. Nonsense mutation
c. Silent mutation
d. Frameshift mutation

82. Southern blotting

a. Was developed in southern U.S.
b. Was named after E.M. Southern
c. Is not useful for detecting gross rearrangements of DNA
d. Cleaves DNA into large fragments

83. Polymerase chain reaction technique for DNA amplification

a. Is slow and cumbersome
b. Can be used to detect nucleotide sequences of infectious agents
c. Is not very specific
d. Must be performed on a fresh whole blood sample

84. Sickle cell anemia

a. Is due to a single base change in the gene that codes for the β chain of hemo-globin
b. Is an example of aneuploidy
c. Involves substitution of glutamic acid for valine in the sixth amino acid position
d. Is inherited as an X-linked recessive disorder

85. Anticipation refers to

a. Waiting for a disease to manifest itself in an individual such as in Huntington's chorea
b. Worsening of a disease phenotype over generations within a family
c. Birth of a fetus with positive prenatal tests for genetic abnormalities
d. Expression of a premutation

86. Which method is used to detect unique genomic DNA fragments from an individual starting with DNA from peripheral leukocytes?

a. Northern blot
b. Southern blot
c. Eastern blot
d. Western blot

87. In autosomal recessive genetic disease, the responsible gene must located on

a. The X chromosome
b. The Y chromosome
c. Any one of the 22 autosomes
d. The X chromosome and one autosome
e. Both X and Y chromosomes

88. A key feature of all X-linked inheritance

a. Male offspring of carrier females have 0% chance of being affected
b. Affected males do not transmit the disease to their sons
c. Affected homozygous females occur when any male mates with a carrier female
d. 50% of female offspring of affected males are carriers
e. Vertical distribution occurs

89. Regarding X inactivation

a. It occurs late in embryonic development
b. Each female is a mosaic with about half of her cells expressing the maternal X and half expressing the paternal X
c. The nonfunctional X chromosome cannot be identified
d. There is more methylation of DNA in the activated compared with the inactivated X chromosome

90. A 21-year-old black man comes to your office complaining of joint pains and swelling of both knees of several months duration. He has had frequent similar episodes beginning before he was 10 years old. His father had similar complaints of joint pains and suffered from anemia. However, his mother did not have any of these symptoms and signs. The patient is also anemic. His hemoglobin gene makeup is likely to be

a. AA
b. SA
c. SS
d. CC
e. AC

Genetic Disease

Answers

46. The answer is c. *(McPhee, 2/e, p 6.)* The phenomenon of different phenotypes in individuals with the same genotype is known as variable expressivity. Polymorphism is an allele that is present in 1% or more of the population. Mutation refers to an event such as a nucleotide change, deletion, or insertion that produces a new allele. Fitness refers to the ability of an affected individual to reproduce.

47. The answer is d. *(McPhee, 2/e, p 5.)* Given a set of defined criteria, recognition of the condition in individuals known to carry the mutated gene is described as penetrance. Reduced penetrance is commonly seen in dominantly inherited conditions that have relatively high fitness such as Huntington's disease or polycystic kidney disease.

48. The answer is b. *(McPhee, 2/e, p 5.)* A phenotype is any characteristic that can be described by an observer. HLA type refers to human leukocyte antigens that are coded by chromosome 6 and are especially important for transplant candidates. Haplotype refers to a set of closely linked alleles that are not easily separated by recombination. Mutation refers to an event such as a nucleotide change, deletion, or insertion that produces a new allele.

49. The answer is a. *(McPhee, 2/e, p 6.)* In males, only one copy of a mutant recessive gene on the X chromosome is sufficient to cause the genetic disease. Females, on the other hand, require two copies of the recessive gene. If this had been a dominantly inherited condition, chances are that at least one of his sisters would be affected.

50. The answer is b. *(McPhee, 2/e, p 13.)* Genetic heterogeneity is defined as a situation in which mutations of different genes produce similar or identical phenotypes. Gonadal mosaicism refers to mutation affecting some of the germ cells (sperm or eggs). Allelic heterogeneity refers to the state in which multiple alleles at a single locus can produce a disease phenotype or phenotypes.

51. The answer is d. *(McPhee, 2/e, p 17.)* A mutant allele that causes death in utero has low fitness. One in which the affected individual lives to reproductive age and allows the individual to pass on the mutant allele has high fitness.

52. The answer is c. *(McPhee, 2/e, p 18.)* When heterozygotes for a disease have a selective advantage compared with homozygous nonaffected individuals, this is called heterozygote advantage. This may account for the high incidence of certain mutant alleles in a population. One example is the high incidence of sickle cell anemia in persons of African descent. The heterozygous state for sickle cell anemia confers protection against malaria and offers a survival advantage.

53. The answer is a. *(McPhee, 2/e, p 6.)* Hypermorphic mutations cause a gain of function. Neomorphic mutations cause the acquisition of a new property. Amorphic mutations cause a complete loss of function. Hypomorphic mutations cause a partial loss of function.

54. The answer is c. *(McPhee, 2/e, p 7.)* Semidominant inheritance probably occurs in most dominantly inherited conditions, but homozygous mutant individuals are rarely observed. One example is when two people with achondroplasia have children. They have a 25% chance of producing a homozygous offspring. Unfortunately, these children usually die in the perinatal period.

55. The answer is c. *(McPhee, 2/e, p 7.)* Cystic fibrosis is inherited as an autosomal recessive disorder that derives from multiple mutations of a gene residing on chromosome 7. It occurs most frequently in whites (1 in 3000 live births). It can cause exocrine problems with the pancreas gland. The mutation responsible for cystic fibrosis most commonly is a deletion of 3 base pairs that code for phenylanaline at amino acid position 508 of the cystic fibrosis transmembrane regulator (CFTR), which functions as a chloride ion channel and other ion channels regulator.

56. The answer is a. *(McPhee, 2/e, p 7.)* About 50% of cases of neurofibromatosis are due to new mutations. Hypermorphism is a mutation that produces an increase in function. A dominant negative mutation gives rise to a protein that interferes with the function of the normal allele. One copy of the dominant negative allele has the same effect as two copies of the allele. This effect is called antimorphic.

57. The answer is b. *(McPhee, 2/e, p 7.)* Duchenne's muscular dystrophy is an X-linked recessive disorder. The patient's mother carries one copy of the recessive gene. It is not expressed in the patient's sisters who may also carry one copy of the recessive gene. Because women possess two X chromosomes, the terms X-linked dominant and X-linked recessive apply only to women. Men, because they possess only one X chromosome, will likely express the full phenotype irrespective of whether the mutation is a dominant or recessive allele in women.

58. The answer is c. *(McPhee, 2/e, p 8.)* Atherosclerosis is believed to be multifactorial. The effects of both genes and the environment play a role in its etiology. The other disorders listed are all single gene disorders.

59. The answer is a. *(McPhee, 2/e, p 9.)* Type I osteogenesis imperfecta is mild. Type II is severe and usually lethal in the perinatal period. Type III is considered progressive and deforming. Type IV is deforming, but with normal scleras.

60. The answer is b. *(McPhee, 2/e, p 9.)* Wormian bones are isolated islands of mineralization in the skull. Type II osteogenesis imperfecta usually results in death in infancy.

61. The answer is c. *(McPhee, 2/e, p 14.)* X-linked disorders are passed on from mother to son. Males are affected more than females in this disorder. One-third of carrier females have a significant degree of mental retardation; 20% of carrier males are nonpenetrant and manifest no signs of the disorder. The mutation involves a highly repetitive area of DNA. Fragile X, the most common cause of inherited mental retardation, results from a trinucleotide repeat expansion of CGG or CCG.

62. The answer is c. *(McPhee, 2/e, p 16.)* CpG islands are several hundred base pairs in length. They have many potential sites for DNA methylation. The CpG island at Xq27.3, the fragile site, is normally unmethylated in male cells, but methylated on one of the two X chromosomes in female cells. The CpG island at Xq27.3 is methylated in affected males and is methylated on both X chromosomes of affected females.

63. The answer is a. *(McPhee, 2/e, p 16.)* Patients with CGG repeat segments of greater than 200 show the fragile X-associated mental retardation syndrome. The fact that in an individual, the actual number of repeats can vary from cell to cell is called genetic mosaicism. Genetic anticipation is shown when a phenotype for a disease is more severe in successive generations. Fitness is the ability of affected individuals to reach the reproductive age and transmit the mutation to offspring. Dosage compensation is the mechanism by which a difference in gene dosage between two cells is equalized. For example, in XX cells, one of the X chromosomes is inactivated, thereby providing a genetic dosage equal to an XY cell.

64. The answer is d. *(McPhee, 2/e, pp 16–17.)* The family mental retardation (FMR1) protein is normally expressed in brain and testes. It is encoded by the *FMR1* gene. Amplification of the CGG region to a repeat number greater than 200 causes methylation of the CpG island and prevents the FMR1 protein from being expressed. This defect is sufficient to cause the fragile X-associated mental retardation syndrome.

65. The answer is a. *(McPhee, 2/e, p 17.)* A premutation allele transmitted by a female expands to a full mutation with a likelihood proportionate to the length of the premutation. Premutation alleles with a repeat number between 52 and 60 rarely expand to a full mutation, whereas those with a repeat number greater than 90 nearly always expand. A premutation allele transmitted by a male rarely if ever expands to a full mutation regardless of the length of the repeat number. A premutation does not cause a change in phenotype. Carrier males have the mutation in their genes. About 20% of carrier males do not show evidence of the disease.

66. The answer is c. *(McPhee, 2/e, p 17.)* Spinocerebellar ataxia 1, spinobulbar muscular atrophy, and Huntington's disease are caused by expansion of a $(5'\text{-CAG-}3')_n$ repeat rather than the $(5'\text{-CFF-}3')_n$ repeat seen in fragile X. The first three diseases involve synthesis of a protein with an expanded polyglutamine region rather than failure to synthesize a normal protein as in fragile X-associated mental retardation syndrome. Only fragile X involves the *FMR1* gene mutation.

67. The answer is b. (*Cecil, 20/e, p 134.*) One copy of the allele is sufficient to produce the phenotype in dominant inheritance. In recessive inheritance, two copies of the allele are necessary to produce the phenotype. An offspring with one parent having the dominant allele has a 50% chance of inheriting the allele. An offspring with both parents having the dominant allele has a 75% chance of inheriting the gene.

68. The answer is b. (*Fauci, 14e, pp 366–367.*) The human genome contains about 50,000 to 100,000 genes. Genes comprise linear strands of DNA that, together with the proteins of chromatin, make up the chromosomes.

69. The answer is c. (*Fauci, 14e, pp 379–380 and 2120–2121.*) Klinefelter's syndrome is a chromosomal disorder and the most frequent major abnormality of sexual differentiation. The chromosome complement is 47,XXY or 46XY/47,XXY. Hemochromatosis and cystic fibrosis are monogenic autosomal recessive disorders, and hemophilia and fragile X are X-linked disorders. Fragile X results from a trinucleotide repeat expansion of CGG or CCG.

70. The answer is a. (*McPhee, 2/e, pp 18–20.*) Women over 35 years of age are at increased risk of giving birth to a child with Down's syndrome. However, screening programs for mothers over age 35 detect most Down's syndrome pregnancies in women of this age group. Because of this fact and the lower total numbers of births to women over age 35, most children with Down's syndrome are born to women under age 35. Individuals with Down's syndrome have statures two to three standard deviations below the average. Weight in affected individuals is mildly increased compared with the general population.

71. The answer is b. (*McPhee, 2/e, p 20.*) Survival depends on the presence or absence of congenital heart disease. Of those with heart disease, 60% survive to age 10 and 50% to age 30. Premature onset of Alzheimer's disease neuropathic changes is present in 100% of affected individuals by age 35. Frank dementia, however, is not detectable in all of these patients and may not play a large role in mortality.

72. The answer is c. (*McPhee, 2/e, p 20.*) It is of interest that both maternal and paternal nondysjunction events are associated with advanced maternal age. It is possible to use molecular markers to tell whether the extra chromosome came from the mother or the father. In studies using these markers, it was found that 75% of the extra chromosome 21 came from the mother and 75% of the nondysjunction events occurred during meiosis I.

73. The answer is a. *(Fauci, 14e, pp 2198–2199.)* Phenylketonuria must be treated before the child is 3 weeks old. Some children may exhibit modest CNS dysfunction with more deleterious mutations or excessive protein intake. Women who have the disease may bear children with congenital anomalies due to maternal transfer of elevated levels of phenylketonuria to the fetus.

74. The answer is c. *(McPhee, 2/e, p 24.)* Newborn screening for PKU is done at 24 to 72 h after birth. The diagnosis is confirmed in about 1% of those screened. The false-negative rate is 1:70. These children are picked up later when they exhibit developmental delays or seizures. Phenylketonuria has a prevalence of 1:10,000.

75. The answer is a. *(McPhee, 2/e, p 24.)* Infants with phenylketonuria are fed a semisynthetic formula low in phenylalanine. This formula can be combined with regular breast feeding. Because phenylalanine is an essential amino acid, infants do require a minimal amount of phenylalanine in their diet. Dietary restriction should be continued indefinitely because even adults with hyperphenylalaninemia develop neuropsychologic and cognitive deficits.

76. The answer is b. *(McPhee, 2/e, p 24.)* The neurologic defects of phenylketonuria are due primarily to phenylalanine itself and not the metabolites. Phenylalanine has a direct effect on energy production, protein synthesis, and neurotransmitter homeostasis. It causes decreased transport of neutral amino acids across the blood-brain barrier. Phenylalanine hydroxylase, which converts phenylalanine to tyrosine, is decreased in action.

77. The answer is b. *(Fauci, 14/e, pp 2195–2198.)* Phenylalanine competitively inhibits tyrosinase and, together with the reduced availability of tyrosine, a melanin precursor, results in the hypopigmentation of hair and skin.

A defect in histidine ammonia lysase occurs in histidinemia with hearing and speech deficits; a defect in cystathionase occurs in cystathioninuria; a defect in sarcosine dehydrogenase occurs in sarcosinemia; and a defect in 4-hydroxyphenylpyruvate dioxygenase occurs in tyrosinemia type III.

78. The answer is b. (*McPhee, 2/e, p 27.*) In phenylketonuria, there is a deficiency in the end products of phenylalanine metabolism, which are catecholamines and neurotransmitters. There is also a buildup of the substrate phenylalanine, which has its own adverse effects.

79. The answer is b. (*Harrison, 14/e, p 366.*) The centimorgan is a measure of genetic distance that reflects the probability of crossover between two loci during meiosis. The human genome is composed of approximately 3000 centimorgans in recombination distance. One centimorgan approximates a 1% chance of crossover during meiosis. The average chromosome contains about 130 centimorgans of genetic material.

80. The answer is d. (*Harrison, 14/e, p 367.*) The likelihood of two parents producing two offspring with identical chromosomes (other than by twinning) is 2^{23} or 1 in 8.4 million.

81. The answer is a. (*Harrison, 14/e, p 369.*) A missense mutation is one in which the base replacement changes the codon for one amino acid to another. A nonsense mutation is one in which the base replacement changes the codon to one of the termination codons. A silent mutation is one in which the base replacement does not lead to a change in the amino acid but only to the substitution of a different codon for the same amino acid. A frameshift mutation is one in which deletion or insertion of one or two bases occurs in a coding region and causes every codon distal to the mutation in the same gene to be read in the wrong triplet frame.

82. The answer is b. (*Harrison, 14/e, p 372.*) Southern blotting was named after E.M. Southern. It is a technique for analyzing DNA where DNA is cleaved into small fragments, fractionated by electrophoreses onto agarose gels, and processed so that specific sequences can be identified. Southern blotting can detect gross rearrangements in DNA and some point mutations.

83. The answer is b. *(Harrison, 14/e, p 372.)* Polymerase chain reaction (PCR) is a technique for amplifying DNA. It can be performed on a fresh blood sample or isolated from dried blood filters, mouthwash, or even old tissue sections. One use is in detecting nucleotide sequences of infectious agents. PCR is a rapid technique that takes a single day. It is automated and extremely specific.

84. The answer is a. *(Harrison, 14/e, p 377.)* Sickle cell anemia is due to a single base change in the gene that codes for the β chain of hemoglobin. The change causes substitution of valine for glutamic acid in the sixth amino acid position in the protein sequence of the β chain. It is inherited as an autosomal recessive disorder. Aneuploidy refers to an abnormal number of chromosomes such as that seen in trisomy 21.

85. The answer is b. *(Harrison, 14/e, p 381.)* In genetics, anticipation refers to the worsening of a disease phenotype over generations within a family. The phenomenon of anticipation is due to increasing size of repeats in premutations that cause earlier onset of disease or a more severe phenotype. The mere presence of premutations does not cause changes in phenotype.

86. The answer is b. *(Harrison, 14/e, p 372.)* This is the definition of Southern blot. Southern blot, named after E.M. Southern, who developed it, is an electrophoresis procedure for separating and identifying DNA. The sensitivity of a Southern blot can be increased by treating whole genomic DNA with restriction endonucleases to produce small fragments that can be separated on an agar gel and identified, e.g., by nucleic acid hybridization. Northern blot is an electrophoresis procedure that starts with RNA and can be used to detect the absence or presence of a particular mRNA. Western blot or immunoblot is an electrophoresis procedure for separation of proteins; the separated proteins can be identified by immunologic procedures, e.g., binding to a radioactive antibody and exposure to a radiographic film for localizing radioactivity.

87. The answer is c. *(Harrison, 14/e, p 383.)* In autosomal recessive disease, males and females are affected in equal proportions so that the gene must be located on any one of the autosomes. Conversely, it cannot be located on the X or Y chromosomes.

88. The answer is b. *(Harrison, 14/e, p 385.)* In X-linked inheritance, male-to-male transmission is absent because the male contributes the Y chromosome to his son and not the X chromosome. All female offspring of affected males are carriers, male offspring of female carriers have a 50% chance of being affected, transmission tends to be oblique and not vertical, and affected homozygous females occur only when an affected male mates with a carrier female.

89. The answer is b. *(Harrison, 14/e, p 386.)* X inactivation occurs early in embryonic development. Because the X chromosome that is selected for inactivation occurs independently and randomly in each cell, it would be expected that females are mosaic with about half of their cells expressing the maternal X and half expressing the paternal X. The nonfunctional X chromosome can be identified as a condensed clump of chromatin called a Barr body. There is more methylation of DNA in the inactivated X chromosome compared with the activated X chromosome.

90. The answer is c. *(Harrison, 14/e, p 648.)* The young man is homozygous SS and exhibits the signs and symptoms of sickle cell disease. Because his father shows the same symptoms and signs, he is likely to be SS also. The mother, who is asymptomatic, is likely heterozygous AS or sickle cell trait, which is a very mild form, mainly with signs and symptoms, as is heterozygous AC. Homozygous CC also is very mild with minimal anemia but not any joint pains or swelling of the joints.

Neoplasia and Blood Disorders

Questions

DIRECTIONS: Each item below contains a question or incomplete statement followed by suggested responses. Select the **one best** response to each question.

91. A 48-year-old white woman has what she believes is a suspicious lump in her breast, but a mammogram does not reveal any suspicious lesions. Truthful statements concerning potential pitfalls in management and diagnosis include

a. Assuming that mammography is "diagnostic"
b. Assuming that a radiographic lesion seen on mammography is the same as a palpable lesion
c. Letting a negative or nonsuspicious mammogram influence the judgment of whether a palpable mass needs to be biopsied
d. Assuming that a benign aspiration cytology is definitive

92. A 55-year-old man has lung cancer in the right middle lobe. Which paraneoplastic syndrome is associated with GHRH secretion and lung cancer?

a. Hypocalcemia
b. Hypocortisolemia
c. Hypophosphatemia
d. Acromegaly
e. Gynecomastia

93. A 30-year-old man has pain in the left scrotum. What is currently valid concerning types of tumor?

a. Alpha fetoprotein (AFP) is only elevated in seminomas.
b. The half-life of AFP is 24 to 36 h.
c. Lactate dehydrogenase (LDH) is an important marker to follow tumor progression or regression.
d. Human chorionic gonadotropin-β subunit (β-hCG) is only elevated in seminoma.

94. In a patient with multiple enlarged lymph nodes, which should be biopsied?

a. Groin nodes
b. Nodes in the axilla
c. Superficial cervical nodes
d. Periaortic lymph node with CT guidance

95. The etiology of chronic lymphocytic leukemia (CLL) is

a. Due to radiation
b. Due to a retrovirus
c. A familial disease
d. Unknown

96. Which of the following is not a major example of inherited susceptibility to cancer?

a. Li-Fraumeni syndrome
b. Familial polyposis coli
c. Familial retinoblastosis
d. Peutz-Jeghers syndrome

97. A 22-year-old man comes to the emergency room of your hospital because he has a diffuse, erythematous rash involving nearly all of his body. His total WBC count is greater than 100,000 cells/mm^3. He also complains of bone pain, severe irritability, weakness, fatigue, nausea and vomiting, constipation, photophobia, and polyuria. His electrocardiogram (ECG) shows shortening of the QT interval, prolongation of the PR interval, and nonspecific T wave changes. The most likely cause of his symptoms is

a. Hypercalcemia
b. Hypocalcemia
c. Hypophosphatemia
d. Hyperkalemia

98. A 45-year-old white man with a limited small cell lung cancer presents to the emergency room of a local hospital and exhibits agitation and confusion, ataxia, nystagmus, peripheral sensory loss, and generalized weakness. The most likely etiology of this disorder is

a. Hypercalcemia
b. Paraneoplastic syndrome
c. Cerebral vascular accident
d. Myasthenia gravis

99. A 52-year-old white woman with breast cancer receiving adjuvant therapy presents with back pain that intensifies on movement and pain over the L1 vertebral body when she coughs and that radiates down her left lower extremity to her leg and foot. The most likely etiology of this disorder is

a. Paraneoplastic disorder
b. Trauma to the lumbar disk
c. Muscular spasm of the intercostal muscles
d. Possible spinal cord compression

100. In the aforementioned patient, the most effective initial treatment is

a. Intravenous Decadron (dexamethasone)
b. Orthopedic consultation
c. Physical therapy techniques
d. Intravenous narcotics

101. A 66-year-old white woman with a known history of small cell lung cancer comes to your office because of engorgement of her neck veins on the right side and over her chest wall. She also has cyanosis of the extremities, facial edema, and difficulty with her mentation. Her diagnosis is most likely

a. Congestive heart failure
b. Lymphatic obstruction of the upper body
c. Superior vena cava syndrome
d. Deep venous thrombosis

102. The multistep theory of carcinogenesis can be applied to what form of cancer?

a. Head and neck cancer
b. Breast cancer
c. Lung cancer
d. Colorectal cancer

103. Platelet production (thrombopoiesis) is affected by more than one cytokine. Which of the following sets seems to be the most important in platelet development?

a. IL-3, granulocyte colony-stimulating factor (G-CSF), and granulocytemacrophage colony-stimulating factor (GM-CSF)
b. IL-4, IL-6, and thrombopoietin
c. Erythropoietin, thrombopoietin, and IL-6
d. IL-6 and thrombopoietin
e. IL-3, IL-4, and IL-6

104. Which of the following factors complexes with factor VIII, which is activated to factor VIIIa when released from the complex?

a. Factor XIII
b. High molecular weight kininogen
c. Von Willebrand factor (vWF)
d. Thromboplastin
e. Plasminogen

105. Which of the following factors depends on platelets for synthesis?

a. Factor II (prothrombin)
b. Factor VII (proconvertin)
c. Protein S
d. Factor XIII (fibrin-stabilizing factor)
e. Factor X (Stuart-Prower factor)

106. Which of the following causes of anemia is associated with microcytosis?

a. Folic acid deficiency
b. Therapy with zidovudine (AZT)
c. Hypothyroidism
d. Alcohol
e. Thalassemia

107. Which of the following causes of an elevated hemoglobin concentration in the blood is characterized by a LOW level of erythropoietin in the blood?

a. Chronic tobacco smoking
b. Dwelling at high altitudes, such as in the Andes
c. Erythrocytosis associated with renal tumors
d. Primary polycythemia (polycythemia vera)
e. Erythrocytosis secondary to chronic pulmonary insufficiency

108. Which of the following causes a leukocytosis without an increase in the number of circulating polymorphonuclear neutrophil leukocytes?

a. Acute infection
b. Release of epinephrine
c. Tissue necrosis
d. Myelocytic leukemia
e. Collagen vascular disease

109. In a typical case of iron deficiency, which of the following molecular forms that contains or can bind to iron increases in the patient's serum?

a. Hemoglobin
b. Ferritin
c. Hemosiderin
d. Myoglobin
e. Transferrin

110. Which of the following disorders is associated with thrombocytosis?

a. Disseminated intravascular coagulation
b. A plastic anemia
c. Postsplenectomy
d. Hypersplenism
e. Prosthetic valves

111. A 47-year-old man walks into the emergency room because of feeling very weak, tired, short of breath, and dizzy. He has numbness and tingling of his fingers. He appears pale and sallow. On examination, his heart rate is 132. His sclerae and nailbeds are pale. His heart is enlarged and he has dependent edema of his ankles. Laboratory findings include a negative Coombs' test and a hemoglobin of 4 g/dL. The likely diagnosis is

a. Traumatic hemolytic anemia
b. Autoimmune anemia
c. Blood loss
d. Pernicious anemia
e. Iron-deficiency anemia

112. Most drugs induce thrombocytopenia by which mechanism?

a. Marrow-depressing effect
b. Directly cytotoxic of platelets
c. Depress megakaryoctye production
d. Immune response in which the platelet is damaged by complement activation
e. Impair megakaryoctye production

113. Which of the following statements related to circulating erythrocytes (red cells) is untrue?

a. The nuclei of the precursor cells to erythrocytes are extruded from their cells shortly before the red cells leave the bone marrow. Consequently, the presence of nucleated red cells in the peripheral blood should be regarded as abnormal and may indicate an underlying disease state.
b. In a thin blood smear stained with Romanowsky's stain (such as Wright's stain), the youngest cells (reticulocytes) can be recognized by a blue coloration (basophilia) as different from most of the red cells present.
c. The average diameter of erythrocytes is about 8 μm; consequently, they cannot flow through the smaller capillaries that have a diameter of 2 to 4 μm.
d. The protein of hemoglobin, which is the principal constituent of the red cell contents, is in tetrameric form, with two α and two β subunits.
e. The iron atom of the hemoglobin molecule, which is essential to its function of carrying oxygen, is an intrinsic part of the heme complex attached to each subunit of protein.

114. Which of the following statements concerning the relationship of the neutrophil polymorphonuclear leukocyte (PMN) to infection with bacterial pathogens is incorrect?

a. The principal functions of the PMN are expressed in the tissues and not usually in the bloodstream, which is simply the transport path of the cells to their required site of action.
b. The cytoplasmic granules of PMN are essentially inert, but metabolically have only a vegetative role in maintaining cell viability.
c. When the cell numbers of PMN are reduced significantly, the probability of severe bacterial infection can be greatly increased.
d. The average duration of the period of circulation of PMN after entering the bloodstream is about 6 to 8 h.
e. An increasing need for PMN produced by infection is met in part by large numbers of immature cells (especially band cells) being released from the marrow pool into the bloodstream.

115. Which pathologic cells in a stained blood film have appearances very similar to those of normal mature white cells or their precursors?

a. Chronic lymphocytic leukemia (B cell type)
b. Chronic myelocytic leukemia
c. Lymphoblastic leukemia
d. Hodgkin's disease
e. Non-Hodgkin's disease

116. On karyotyping, a well-defined chromosomal abnormality is pathognomonic of which condition?

a. Chronic lymphocytic leukemia (B cell type)
b. Chronic myelocytic leukemia
c. Lymphoblastic leukemia
d. Hodgkin's disease
e. Non-Hodgkin's disease

117. Which condition customarily terminates by transition to a blast cell phase with similarities to acute leukemia?

a. Chronic lymphocytic leukemia (B cell type)
b. Chronic myelocytic leukemia
c. Lymphoblastic leukemia
d. Hodgkin's disease
e. Non-Hodgkin's disease

118. The principal complication of which condition is susceptibility to infection?

a. Chronic lymphocytic leukemia (B cell type)
b. Chronic myelocytic leukemia
c. Lymphoblastic leukemia
d. Hodgkin's disease
e. Non-Hodgkin's disease

119. Which disorder presents mainly as a localized new mass or group of superficial lymph nodes?

a. Chronic lymphocytic leukemia (B cell type)
b. Chronic myelocytic leukemia
c. Lymphoblastic leukemia
d. Hodgkin's disease
e. Non-Hodgkin's disease

120. Which mechanism is responsible for thrombocytopenia in vitamin B_{12} deficiency?

a. Decreased production
b. Maldistribution
c. Accelerated destruction
d. Decreased survival
e. Inherited

121. Which mechanism is responsible for thrombocytopenia in disseminated intravascular coagulation (DIC)?

a. Decreased production
b. Maldistribution
c. Accelerated destruction
d. Decreased survival
e. Inherited

122. Which mechanism is responsible for thrombocytopenia in immune (idiopathic) thrombocytopenic purpura (ITP)?

a. Decreased production
b. Maldistribution
c. Accelerated destruction
d. Decreased survival
e. Inherited

123. Which mechanism is responsible for thrombocytopenia in any increase in spleen size?

a. Decreased production
b. Maldistribution
c. Accelerated destruction
d. Decreased survival
e. Inherited

124. Which mechanism is responsible for thrombocytopenia in thrombotic thrombocytopenic purpura (TTP)?

a. Decreased production
b. Maldistribution
c. Accelerated destruction
d. Decreased survival
e. Inherited

125. Which mechanism is responsible for thrombocytopenia in von Willebrand's syndrome?

a. Decreased production
b. Maldistribution
c. Accelerated destruction
d. Decreased survival
e. Inherited

126. Which is a protein cofactor that exposes the inactivation site of activated coagulation factor V, which can then be cleaved by a protease?

a. Protein C
b. Protein S
c. Antithrombin III (ATIII)
d. Plasminogen
e. Prekallikrein

127. Which is a factor capable of inhibiting the serine protease factors II, IX, X, XI, and XII, a process accelerated by heparin or similar molecules.

a. Protein C
b. Protein S
c. Antithrombin III (ATIII)
d. Plasminogen
e. Prekallikrein

128. Which is a vitamin K–dependent factor, activated in the presence of thrombin to cleave activated factors V and VIII.

a. Protein C
b. Protein S
c. Antithrombin III (ATIII)
d. Plasminogen
e. Prekallikrein

Neoplasia and Blood Disorders

Answers

91. The answer is c. *(Fauci, 14/e, p 363.)* Any suspicious palpable mass should be biopsied despite a negative mammogram. Negative mammograms can occur in 10 to 15% of instances of a palpable breast mass.

92. The answer is d. *(Fauci, 14/e, p 620.)* Ectopic acromegaly is a paraneoplastic endocrine disorder related to small cell lung cancer and secretion of growth hormone–releasing hormone (GHRH). Hypercalcemia is a paraneoplastic endocrine syndrome associated with non-small cell cancers which is caused by secretion of parathyroid hormone–related peptides (PTHrP); hypercortisolism caused by ACTH release occurs with small cell lung cancers, and cellular release of phosphorus causes hyperphosphatemia associated with lung cancer; gynecomastia caused by human chorionic gonadotropin secretion (hCG) also occurs with lung cancers.

93. The answer is c. *(Fauci, 14/e, p 603.)* LDH is an important marker to follow in any germ cell tumor. AFP elevation is seen only in nonseminoma, whereas β-hCG is seen in both nonseminoma and seminoma. The half-life of AFP is 5 to 7 days.

94. The answer is c. *(Fauci, 14/e, pp 346 and 347.)* Cervical nodes are more likely to yield an etiology of disease than those in the axillae and supraclavicular region. Nodes in the inguinal/femoral (groin) area much less often provide diagnosis of disease because they often are nonspecifically enlarged because of repeated infections of the lower extremities.

95. The answer is d. *(Fauci, 14/e, p 699.)* Chronic lymphocytic leukemia (CLL), a common chronic leukemia, has no known etiology. B cell CLL is the most common chronic leukemia/lymphoma. Often it presents as an asymptomatic lymphocytosis in patients about 60 years old.

96. The answer is d. *(Fauci, 14/e, p 513.)* Li-Fraumeni syndrome, familial polyposis coli, and familial retinoblastosis are known genetic disorders associated with familial malignancies. Peutz-Jeghers syndrome, a familial disorder of multiple gastrointestinal polyps, rarely occurs as a familial cancer disorder.

97. The answer is a. *(Fauci, 14/e, pp 618–619.)* Hypercalcemia of malignancy is the most common paraneoplastic syndrome. It accounts for about 40% of all hypercalcemia. The signs and symptoms of hypercalcemia include bone pain, irritability, weakness, fatigue, constipation, nausea, and vomiting, as this patient manifests. Symptoms begin at a serum calcium of about 2.6 mmol/L. Hypercalcemia of malignancy is common in cancers with squamous cell histology.

98. The answer is b. *(Fauci, 14/e, pp 618–622.)* The paraneoplastic syndromes include endocrine syndromes and hematologic syndromes. The paraneoplastic endocrine syndromes include hypercalcemia of malignancy, inappropriate vasopressin secretion (SIADH), Cushing's syndrome, acromegaly, and gynecomastia. The paraneoplastic hematologic disorders include erythrocytosis, granulocytosis, thrombocytosis, eosinophilia, and thrombophlebitis.

99. The answer is d. *(Fauci, 14/e, pp 628–629.)* Any back pain in a patient with a known history of carcinoma should be evaluated for the possibility of spinal cord compression. It occurs in 5 to 10% of patients with cancer. Lung cancer is the most common primary malignancy causing spinal cord compression. Localized back pain and tenderness are the most common initial complaints.

100. The answer is a. *(Fauci, 14/e, pp 628–629.)* Intravenous Decadron is the choice for initial treatment in this situation because it will decrease swelling of the tumor mass. It may provide some relief of the compression by reducing the edema. It should be given immediately on making the diagnosis.

101. The answer is c. *(Fauci, 14/e, p 627.)* The definitive diagnosis is superior vena cava syndrome until proven otherwise with scans. It means that the superior vena cava is obstructed. Ninety percent of these cases are due to malignant tumors such as carcinoma of the lung, lymphoma, and various metastatic tumors. The findings described in this patient are not due to the other diagnoses.

102. The answer is d. *(Fauci, 14/e, p 517.)* Colon cancer is one cancer in which the multistep theory of carcinogenesis has been studied. In the multistep theory, the cancer develops from multiple somatic mutational steps that change normal epithelium to adenoma to carcinoma. An accumulation of somatic mutations is necessary for cancer to develop.

103. The answer is d. *(McPhee, 2/e, pp 99–100.)* Platelet production is stimulated by multiple cytokines, the most important being IL-6 and the peptide thrombopoietin. IL-3, IL-6, and GM-CSF also affect megakaryocytes, whereas erythropoietin and G-CSF are almost exclusively related to erythropoiesis and granulocyte production, respectively. IL-4 is also predominantly granulocyte related.

104. The answer is c. *(McPhee, 2/e, pp 104–105; Fauci, 14/e, pp 339–342.)* VWF complexes with factor VIII, which is activated by release from the complex to produce factor VIIIa. Together with factor IXa, calcium, and platelet phospholipid, factor VIIIa activates factor X. Factor XIII is activated to XIIIa by thrombin and improves the tensile properties of fibrin by chemical cross-linking. High molecular weight kininogen is the activator of factor XII. Thromboplastin is the lipid-rich protein material released on tissue injury that activates factor VII. Plasminogen is the precursor of plasmin, which is the serum protease that cleaves fibrin.

105. The answer is d. *(McPhee, 2/e, p 104; Fauci, 14/e, p 739.)* Factor XIII is produced by platelets. Factors II, VII, IX, and X are all dependent for synthesis on γ-carboxylase, a liver enzyme dependent on vitamin K. The two anticoagulant proteins S and C are also vitamin K dependent. Vitamin K is a necessary cofactor in the posttranslational synthesis of γ-carboxyglutamic acid groups in precursors of these factors.

106. The answer is e. *(McPhee, 2/e, p 105; Fauci, 14/e, pp 338 and 643.)* Microcytic anemia results from abnormal hemoglobin production of the quantity of molecules or the type, as in thalassemia. Macrocytic anemia results either from abnormal nuclear maturation (nuclear–cytoplasmic asynchrony) with megaloblastic changes in the bone marrow precursor cells or a high proportion of reticulocytes in the red cell population. The causes of abnormal nuclear maturation include vitamin B_{12} deficiency, folic acid deficiency, drugs that interfere with DNA synthesis, and alcohol. A high proportion of reticulocytes in the red cell population will also increase the average mean volume of red cells, because reticulocytes are larger than more mature red cells. This occurs when there is an active marrow proliferative response in compensation for active red cell destruction (hemolysis) or an active response to therapy for anemia such as vitamin B_{12}.

107. The answer is d. (*McPhee, 2/e, p 105; Fauci, 14/e, pp 679–680.*) The relative hypoxia of the tobacco smoker, the mountain dweller, and the patient with pulmonary insufficiency is a stimulus to erythropoietin production, which results in increased red cell production and circulating red cell mass. Likewise, some tumors, including renal tumors, uterine myomata, and cerebellar hemangiomas, may synthesize erythropoietin. Primary polycythemia is an abnormality of the bone marrow, leading to increased circulating red cell mass and feedback suppression of erythropoietin production.

108. The answer is b. (*McPhee, 2/e, p 106; Fauci, 14/e, pp 352 and 355.*) The leukocytosis associated with release of epinephrine, including conditions of stress (endogenous) and in therapy (exogenous), arises by demargination of neutrophils from the blood vessel walls. The apparent increase in the leukocyte count results from redistribution of the neutrophils, the marginated cells normally flowing close to the periphery of the blood vessels being relocated throughout the full volume of flowing blood. Leukocytosis associated with acute infection, tissue necrosis, myelocytic leukemia, and collagen vascular disease is due to the proliferative stimulus increasing the true numbers of circulating cells.

109. The answer is e. (*McPhee, 2/e, p 109; Fauci, 14/e, pp 337 and 640.*) Transferrin is the principal iron-binding protein present in plasma and carries the greater part of the iron in transport between the gut, storage sites, and the bone marrow. In iron deficiency, the total iron-binding capacity of serum increases as the serum iron falls. The iron-binding capacity is principally dependent on the quantity of transferrin. Hemoglobin and myoglobin contain iron in the oxygen-carrying molecule heme. This binds oxygen reversibly, which permits transport by hemoglobin in red cells and storage by myoglobin in muscle.

110. The answer is c. (*McPhee, 2/e, p 107; Fauci, 14/e, p 683.*) Thrombocytosis occurs in the myeloproliferative disorders (especially essential thrombocythemia), in the hyposplenic states, including postsplenectomy, mainly because of redistribution of the excess platelets normally present in the spleen and anemias. The anemias include iron-deficiency anemia and hemolytic anemias, reflecting the increased proliferative activity of the affected bone marrow. Thrombocytopenia occurs because of decreased production as in aplastic anemia, vitamin B_{12}, and folate deficiencies or because of decreased survival as in hypersplenism, prosthetic valves, and disseminated intravascular coagulation.

111. The answer is d. (*McPhee, 2/e, pp 111–113; Fauci, 14/e, pp 653–659.*) Pernicious anemia, a megaloblastic anemia, results from a complex cascade of events that is autoimmune in origin. Antibodies against gastric parietal cell components and intrinsic factor are common, and antibody-generating B lymphocytes are found in the gastric mucosa. The signs of vitamin B_{12} (cobalamin) deficiency are delayed by the liver storage of cobalamin, provided that the patient's intake has previously been normal. Cobalamin deficiency is almost always due to malabsorption. Normal diets usually provide adequate intake of cobalamin; however, in vegetarians the intake is inadequate. Persons suffering from pernicious anemia can develop very low hemoglobin levels, as low as 4 g/dL, unlike other anemias. Multiple neurologic findings (due to demyelination at first and then axonal degeneration) include numbness and paresthesias, weakness, ataxia, difficulties with mentation, and abnormal deep tendon reflexes and pathological reflexes, high output failure, sallow color are consistent with pernicious anemia. In autoimmune hemolysis, the Coombs' test is positive.

112. The answer is d. (*McPhee, 2/e, pp 117–119; Fauci, 14/e, pp 731 and 744.*) Drugs induce thrombocytopenia by an immune response. The platelet is damaged by complement activation as a consequence of the formation of drug-antibody complexes. The incidence of thrombocytopenia is high in patients treated with heparin. The pathogenesis involves binding of heparin to platelet factor 4 (PF4), and the released heparin–PF4 combination acts as an antigen provoking the production of an IgG antibody. The complex IgG–heparin–PF can bind to platelets by the platelet Fc receptor and lead to thrombocytopenia by destruction of the sensitized platelets in the spleen. However, the complex can also form bridges between platelets and induce aggregation with platelet activation and the potential for thrombus formation. Heparin-induced thrombosis is sometimes known as the "white clot syndrome." Alcohol ingested in large quantities depresses the marrow, and chemotherapeutic drugs are cytotoxic and depress megakaryocyte production.

113. The answer is c. (*McPhee, 2/e, pp 100–101.*) The presence of nucleated red cells in the peripheral blood is abnormal: it may be pathologic as in the leukoerythroblastosis that accompanies bone marrow infiltration, or with extramedullary erythropoiesis as in primary (agnogenic) myeloid metaplasia. Occasionally, it accompanies a brisk therapeutic correction of anemia. The earliest red cells (reticulocytes) still contain some ribosomes, mitochondria, and RNA and appear faintly basophilic (blue) in a Wright's stained blood smear. Hemoglobin is a tetrameric protein, and each subunit is associated with a heme complex containing the iron atom of the molecule, which is related to the locus of the carried oxygen atoms. The red cell is, in fact, normally a highly flexible body, capable of considerable modification of shape in traversing small capillaries. The flexibility may be compromised by increased intracellular viscosity or rigidity of the cell membrane, as in various hemolytic anemias.

114. The answer is b. (*McPhee, 2/e, p 101; Fauci, 14/e, p 351.*) The neutrophils (PMNs) are the predominant form of the WBCs, but their major function is in the tissues where they accumulate at sites of infection or inflammation, after transient passage through the bloodstream. Decreased available numbers (neutropenia) can result in a high incidence of bacterial infections. The granules contain enzymes with bactericidal properties, such as myeloperoxidase and NADPH oxidase.

115–119. The answers are 115: b; 116: b; 117: b; 118: a; 119: d. (*McPhee, 2/e, p 106; Fauci, 14/e, pp 691–694 and 697–699.*) The chronic lymphocytic and myelocytic leukemias are characterized by proliferation of lymphoid and myeloid cells, which are usually present in excessive numbers in the peripheral blood: their appearances in the peripheral blood smear are usually close to those of the related normal forms, although other properties of the cells may be abnormal. Precursor forms are often prominent in myeloid leukemias. A characteristic chromosomal translocation t(9:22) results in the Philadelphia chromosome: although not exclusively restricted to chronic myelocytic leukemia, its presence in a chronic leukemia makes the diagnosis highly probable. The myelocytic leukemia commonly terminates following transition to an accelerated phase with transformation of the principal malignant cell to a blastlike form. The lymphocytic leukemia involves impaired antibody production and other immune functions, resulting in susceptibility to severe infections. Both forms of leukemia lead to increasing accumulation of malignant cells, leading to organ enlargement, especially of the spleen, liver, lymph nodes, and bone marrow. Hodgkin's disease often presents with superficial nodes found as a new mass.

120–125. The answers are 120: a; 121: c; 122: c; 123: b; 124: c; 125: e. (*McPhee, 2/e, p 107; Fauci, 14/e, pp 344 and 730–731.*) Thrombocytopenia is most commonly produced by processes that reduce the survival of circulating platelets significantly below the normal average life span of 10 days. In disseminated intravascular coagulation, activation of the coagulation sequence by infection, release of thromboplastins from malignant cells, hypoxia, or hemorrhage leads to a consumption coagulopathy that depletes the components of coagulation mechanisms, including the platelets. In vitamin B_{12} (cobalamin) deficiency, the number of megakaryocytes in the bone marrow are depleted. In ITP, autoimmune antibodies attack the platelet surface and initiate phagocytosis by attachment to the receptors of macrophages, especially in the spleen. A proportion, often about 10%, of the circulating platelets is normally present in a platelet pool in a normal spleen. With splenic enlargement (splenomegaly), the pool accommodates a higher proportion of the total and reduces the platelet count. Von Willebrand's syndrome is an inherited disorder in which affected persons lack the carrier protein for factor VIII, the von Willebrand factor, and it is necessary for formation of the platelet plug in the coagulation cascade.

126–128. The answers are 126: c; 127: c; 128: a. (*McPhee, 2/e, pp 120–122; Fauci, 14/e, pp 341–342.*) Control of the coagulation system depends in large part on the activity of negative control factors that impede the excessive development of active coagulation. Protein C, which exposes the inactivation site of activated coagulation factor V, is an anticoagulation factor requiring vitamin K for its synthesis. Thrombin generated by the coagulation process and modified by thrombomodulin activates protein C, which cleaves factors Va and VIIIa and inhibits coagulation. Platelet phospholipid, calcium, and a cofactor, protein S, are also required. Antithrombin III (ATIII) is also an inhibitor of coagulation not only of thrombin but of activated IX, X, XI, and XII. It acts by binding to the factor and not by enzymatic action. Its activity is very dependent on its accelerator cofactor, heparin. Activated factor XIII is involved in cross-linking fibrin, and prekallikrein is involved in activating factor XII.

Infectious Disease

Questions

DIRECTIONS: Each item contains a question or incomplete statement followed by suggested responses. Select the **one best** response to each question.

129. Acute bacterial infections of the bone characteristically show which one of the following?

a. Necrotic bone
b. Prolonged clinical course
c. Predominantly mononuclear cells
d. Congested and thrombosed blood vessels
e. Granulation tissue

130. Which one of the following organisms accounts for at least 50% of cases of acute hematogenous and contiguous focus osteomyelitis?

a. Group A streptococci
b. Group B streptococci
c. *Mycoplasma*
d. *S. aureus*
e. *Pseudomonas aeruginosa*

131. Bacteria can infect the skin through accidental or deliberate breaks in it or through the hair follicle. Which one bacteria causes one of several differing infections of the skin including necrotizing fasciitis, erysipelas, impetigo contagiosa, and necrotizing myositis?

a. *Clostridium* spp.
b. *S. pyogenes*
c. *S. aureus*
d. Anaerobic bacteria
e. *Pseudomonas aeruginosa*

132. Which one of the following does not contribute to injection drug users becoming infected?

a. Unsterile injection technique
b. Immune defects induced by drug use
c. Contaminated needles and syringes
d. Nonuse of antibiotics
e. Poor dental hygiene

133. Infective endocarditis frequently occurs in injection drug users. The valve most often involved is

a. Mitral
b. Aortic
c. Tricuspid
d. Pulmonic

134. Which one of the following types of bites is more likely to become infected?

a. Human
b. Dog
c. Cat
d. Rat

135. Among nosocomial (hospital acquired) infections, which one occurs most commonly and also causes the least sequelae?

a. Pneumonia
b. Urinary tract
c. Surgical wound
d. Bacteremia

136. Gram-negative and gram-positive bacteria each possess which one of the following structures?

a. Peptidoglycan
b. Lipopolysaccharide
c. Matrix protein
d. Pili
e. Flagella

137. Which organism is not a likely cause of left-sided infective endo-carditis?

a. *Clostridium* spp.
b. *S. aureus*
c. *Streptococcus viridans*
d. *Enterococcus*
e. *Streptococcus bovis*

138. The subarachnoid space inflammation of bacterial meningitis, which is caused by a gram-negative bacteria, is induced by which one component of the bacteria?

a. Matrix protein
b. Lipopolysaccharide (LPS)
c. Pili
d. Inner membrane
e. Peptidoglycan

139. Which one of the following microorganisms is the most common cause of meningitis in children under 1 month of age?

a. *Neisseria meningitidis*
b. *Streptococcus pneumoniae* (pneumococcus)
c. Gram-negative bacilli
d. Staphylococci
e. *Hemophilus influenzae*

140. Which one of the following microorganisms is the most common cause of community acquired pneumonia?

a. *Mycoplasma pneumoniae*
b. *Streptococcus pneumoniae*
c. *Staphylococcus aureus*
d. *Hemophilus influenzae*
e. *Legionella* spp.

141. Which one of the following microorganisms is not a likely cause of pneumonia among persons with human immunodeficiency virus (HIV) infection and AIDS?

a. *Mycoplasma pneumoniae*
b. *Streptococcus pneumoniae*
c. *Pneumocystis carinii*
d. *Hemophilus influenzae*
e. *Mycobacterium tuberculosis*

142. Which one of the following bacteria is deposited directly into the lower airways?

a. *Mycoplasma pneumoniae*
b. *Streptococcus pneumoniae*
c. *Pneumocystis carinii*
d. *Hemophilus influenzae*
e. *Mycobacterium tuberculosis*

143. Which microorganism is likely to cause pneumonia in a person with late stages of HIV and AIDS?

a. *Legionella* spp.
b. *Pneumocystis carinii*
c. *Chlamydia psittaci*
d. *Klebsiella pneumoniae*
e. *Moraxella catarrhalis*

144. Which microorganism is likely to cause pneumonia in a person who abuses alcohol?

a. *Legionella* spp.
b. *Pneumocystis carinii*
c. *Chlamydia psittaci*
d. *Klebsiella pneumoniae*
e. *Moraxella catarrhalis*

145. Which one of the following microorganisms that cause pneumonia is acquired from exposure to an infected animal?

a. *Legionella* spp.
b. *Pneumocystis carinii*
c. *Chlamydia psittaci*
d. *Klebsiella pneumoniae*
e. *Moraxella catarrhalis*

146. Persons with chronic pulmonary disease are more likely to develop pneumonia due to infection which one of the following pathogens?

a. *Legionella* spp.
b. *Pneumocystis carinii*
c. *Chlamydia psittaci*
d. *Klebsiella pneumoniae*
e. *Moraxella catarrhalis*

147. Which one of the following groups of microorganisms more commonly causes diarrhea in the United States?

a. Bacteria
b. Fungi
c. Protozoa
d. Viruses

148. The single most important bacteria that causes diarrhea worldwide is:

a. *Helicobacter pylori*
b. *Staphylococcus aureus*
c. *Salmonella* spp.
d. *Shigella* spp.
e. *E. coli*

149. In the pathogenesis of acute diarrhea, which microorganism characteristically penetrates intestinal mucosa of the distal small bowel, multiplies in Peyer's patches, and then disseminates by the bloodstream?

a. *Vibrio cholerae*
b. Enterotoxigenic *E. coli*
c. *Salmonella typhi*
d. *Rotavirus*
e. *Clostridium difficile*

150. Which one of the endogenous mediators of sepsis is most likely to be the mediator of shock?

a. Cytokines
b. Endorphins
c. Arachidonic acid metabolites
d. Complement C5a
e. Nitric oxide

151. The principal CD lymphocyte affected in HIV and AIDS is:

a. CD28
b. CD27
c. CD8
d. CD4
e. CD3

152. The destruction of CD4 lymphocytes in HIV and AIDS involves all of the following except which one feature?

a. Direct viral destruction of CD4 lymphocytes
b. Apoptosis
c. Autoimmunity
d. Syncytium formation
e. Bone marrow stimulation

153. Typically HIV progresses from the onset of infection to evidence of immunosuppression over what period of time?

a. 1 to 3 months
b. 1 to 3 years
c. 4 to 5 years
d. 5 to 10 years
e. 11 to 15 years

154. Which one of the following causes a lung infection, the most common opportunistic infection, in HIV-infected persons?

a. Kaposi's sarcoma
b. *Pneumocystis carinii*
c. *Mycobacterium tuberculosis*
d. *Mycobacterium avium complex* (MAC)
e. *Toxoplasma gondii*

155. Which one of the following causes esophagitis, with substernal pain and dysphagia, in HIV-infected persons?

a. *Candida albicans*
b. Cytomegalovirus
c. *Cryptococcus neoformans*
d. *Herpesvirus varicellae*
e. *Cryptosporidium*

156. Which one of the following causes biliary tract infection, including sclerosing cholangitis, in HIV-infected persons?

a. *Candida albicans*
b. Cytomegalovirus
c. *Cryptococcus neoformans*
d. *Herpesvirus varicellae*
e. *Cryptosporidium*

157. Which one of the following causes painful and crusted lesions that follow the path of an intracostal nerve in persons infected with HIV?

a. *Candida albicans*
b. Cytomegalovirus
c. *Cryptococcus neoformans*
d. *Herpesvirus varicellae*
e. *Cryptosporidium*

158. Which one of the following causes headache, seizures, altered mental status, and a space-occupying lesion in persons infected with HIV?

a. Kaposi's sarcoma
b. *Pneumocystis carinii*
c. *Mycobacterium tuberculosis*
d. *Mycobacterium avium complex*
e. *Toxoplasma gondii*

159. Which one of the following causes localized skin lesion or disseminated visceral lesion characterized by mixed cell population that includes vascular endothelial cells in persons infected with HIV?

a. Kaposi's sarcoma
b. *Pneumocystis carinii*
c. *Mycobacterium tuberculosis*
d. *Mycobacterium avium complex*
e. *Toxoplasma gondii*

160. Which one of the following causes retinitis, with patient complaints of blind spots, and retinal hemorrhages and exudates in persons infected with HIV?

a. *Candida albicans*
b. Cytomegalovirus
c. *Cryptococcus neoformans*
d. *Herpesvirus varicellae*
e. *Cryptosporidium*

161. Which one of the following causes a wasting disease and cachexia in persons infected with HIV?

a. Kaposi's sarcoma
b. *Pneumocystis carinii*
c. *Mycobacterium tuberculosis*
d. *Mycobacterium avium complex*
e. *Toxoplasma gondii*

162. A 45-year-old woman veterinarian who is a faculty member at the nearby veterinary school comes to your office with complaints of a flulike syndrome of 9 days' duration including persistent fever for all 9 days, extreme fatigue, and severe headache. She has a dry cough, an increased white count, and thrombocytopenia. Which one of the following is the likely cause of her infection?

a. *Influenzavirus*
b. *Mycoplasma pneumoniae*
c. *Chlamydia psittaci*
d. *Coxiella burnetii*
e. *Chlamydia pneumoniae*

163. Pneumococcal vaccine is

a. Comprised of purified capsular polysaccharides from 23 serotypes
b. Precipitated with alum to improve its antigenicity
c. Inactivated with formaldehyde
d. Prepared by recombinant techniques
e. Revised annually based on the predominant serotypes in the U.S.

164. A 22-year-old college student comes to your office because of a cold and respiratory symptoms of about 12 days' duration that do not seem to be lessening in intensity. He is anorexic and tired. His respiratory rate is 24/min, and he has a cough productive of small amounts of white sputum, but no hemoptysis or pleuritic chest pain. He chest x-ray shows infiltration in the right lower lobe. He has a leukocytosis of 18,000 and his cold agglutinin titer is elevated. The organism that is the likely cause of this illness is

a. *Leptospira*
b. *Influenzavirus*
c. *Mycoplasma pneumoniae*
d. *Legionella* spp.
e. *Coxiella burnetti*

165. In clinical infection with *E. histolytica*, the main finding concerning immunity is

a. Clinical infection induces immunity to recurrent colonization
b. Repeated episodes of colitis are usual
c. Antibody is protective
d. Antibody titers correlate with the length of illness
e. Antibody titers correlate with the severity of disease

166. The recommendation for poliovirus vaccine in infants and children was changed to inactivated vaccine [Salk inactivated vaccine (IPV)] from live attenuated vaccine [Sabin oral vaccine (OPV)] for which reason?

a. Inactivated vaccine is cheaper than attenuated vaccine
b. Injection of vaccine is easier than oral administration
c. The antibody response is more long lasting with inactivated vaccine
d. The chance of vaccine-induced polio illness is unlikely with inactivated vaccine
e. Mothers prefer injections for their children

167. INH prophylaxis is recommended for which person?

a. A man teacher with HIV and a PPD of 4 mm
b. A well man truck driver age 25 years with a PPD of 8 mm
c. A well woman clerk age 45 years with a PPD of 9 mm
d. A well man medical student age 30 years with a PPD of 11 mm
e. A well woman actress age 40 years with a PPD of 12 mm

168. Among intravenous drug abusers, which is most often the source of the pathogens of infective endocarditis?

a. Urine
b. Lungs
c. Gastrointestinal tract
d. Skin
e. Contaminated drugs

169. Which is the best approach to confirm the diagnosis of an acute cytomegalovirus infection (CMV)?

a. Clinically with fever and rash
b. Isolation of the virus from urine
c. Isolation of virus from saliva
d. Isolation of the virus from blood
e. Isolation of virus from stool

170. The complications of severe infections of falciparum malaria can include anemia that is due predominantly to

a. Significant bleeding with disseminated intravascular coagulation
b. Accelerated erythrocyte destruction and removal by the spleen
c. Inadequate iron storage
d. Increased Kuppfer cells in the liver
e. Lactic acidosis

171. Which one feature characterizes cat-scratch disease?

a. 60% of cases occur in adults
b. Fever and rash occur within 3 to 5 days of a cat scratch in most cases
c. Anorexia, malaise, and weight loss are common
d. Painless lymphadenopathy
e. Culture of lymph nodes usually is positive for the infecting organism

172. A 12-year-old boy is brought to your office by his mother because he developed a painless rash on his face and legs. The rash began as red papules and then became vesicular and pustular and finally it coalesced in honeycomb-like crusts. The boy does not have fever, but he does have several insect bites and he is unwashed and dressed in dirty clothes. This rash is likely to be

a. Herpes simplex
b. Shingles
c. Impetigo
d. Scarlet fever
e. Erysipelas

Infectious Disease

Answers

129. The answer is d. *(Fauci, 14e, p 824.)* Acute osteomyelitis shows bacteria, polymorphonuclear leukocytes, and congested and thrombosed blood vessels. Its course is not prolonged, as is the course of chronic osteomyelitis. Necrotic bone, presence of granulation and fibrous tissues, very few bacteria, and the absence of living osteocytes characterize chronic osteomyelitis.

130. The answer is d. *(Fauci, 14e, pp 824–825.)* In acute hematogenous osteomyelitis, *S. aureus* accounts for about 50% of infections, likely as the single organism. In contiguous focus osteomyelitis, *S. aureus* also occurs in more than 50% of cases, except it likely occurs together with other organisms as a polymicrobial infection.

131. The answer is b. *(Fauci, 14e, p 828.)* *S. pyogenes* causes these differing skin infections because they infect the dermis and can spread laterally by the lymphatics to deeper and superficial areas. *Pseudomonas aeruginosa* causes hot tub folliculitis especially in tubs that fail to maintain high water temperature, for example between 37° and 40°C, and sufficient chlorination. *S. aureus* causes bullous impetigo, furunculosis, and pyomyositis. Clostridium species causes gas gangrene.

132. The answer is d. *(Fauci, 14e, p 831.)* Usually, intermittent antibiotic usage by injection drug users alters normal microbial flora, leading to increased risk of infection, and the nonuse of antibiotics would prevent it. All other factors contribute to the increased of infection in injection drug users.

133. The answer is c. *(Fauci, 14e, p 832.)* The tricuspid valve is more frequently involved than the other valves, perhaps because of its nearness to the injection sites. However, in an individual patient any of the heart valves may become infected. Left-sided infective endocarditis usually develops when underlying valvular defect exists.

134. The answer is a. *(Fauci, 14e, p 837.)* Of the common animal bites, human bites more often become infected than other animal bites. They occur as occlusional injuries: actual biting and clenched-fist injuries sustained by striking the teeth of another individual. Infections caused by human bites reflect the multiple microorganisms that can be present in the mouth.

135. The answer is b. *(Fauci, 14e, p 848.)* Urinary tract infections acquired in hospital develop more commonly than any other nosocomial infection and have the fewest severe sequelae. The other nosocomial infections, especially pneumonia and bacteremia, are life threatening and much more difficult to treat and can lead to severe sequelae.

136. The answer is a. *(Fauci, 14e, p 853.)* Gram-positive and gram-negative bacteria each have a peptidoglycan layer. All other structures are features of gram-negative bacteria only.

137. The answer is a. *(Fauci, 14e, pp 785–786.)* The most common bacteria causing infective endocarditis of the left side of the heart are viridans streptococci (including *Streptococcus sanguis, Streptococcus mutans,* and *Streptococcus mitis*), less often *Streptococcus bovis* and other streptococci, *S. aureus* and *Enterococcus. Clostridium* spp. and other fungi are pathogens of endocarditis in persons who are injection drug abusers, but rarely in other persons. *S. aureus* also is common in injection drug users, and then it infects the right side of the heart.

138. The answer is b. *(Fauci, 14e, p 2422.)* The pathogenesis of meningitis involves subarachnoid space inflammation caused by the invading bacterial pathogen. Individual component(s) of the bacteria induce subarachnoid space inflammation. In the case of the gram-negative bacteria, the lipopolysaccharide (LPS or endotoxin) induces subarachnoid space inflammation, but in the pneumococcus, it's the cell wall components, namely, teichoic acid and peptidoglycan. Both bacteria do this through the release of inflammatory mediators.

139. The answer is c. *(Fauci, 14e, p 2419.)* Among children 1 month of age and younger, the gram-negative bacilli, mainly *E. coli* and other enteric bacilli, are the most common cause of meningitis. Group B streptococci and *Listeria monocytogenes* also cause meningitis in this age of group of children, but not as often as do the gram-negative bacilli. Group B streptococci septic infections that occur very early do so as a result of spread of the organism to the newborn from the maternal genital tract. *N. meningitidis* is a common cause of meningitis in children older than 1 month of age, and among older children, adolescents, and adults, *N. meningitidis* and *S. pneumoniae* are the two most common pathogens of meningitis. *H. influenzae* is a common cause of meningitis among older children and adolescents.

140. The answer is b. (*McPhee, 2e, p 64.*) *S. pneumoniae* is the most common cause of community acquired pneumonia, accounting for about two-thirds of pneumonias, especially among adults. *Mycoplasma pneumoniae* occurs mainly in young adults during the second and third decades. *H. influenzae* is a frequent cause of community acquired, but not the most frequent. *S. aureus* and *Legionella* spp. are minor causes of community acquired pneumonia.

141. The answer is a. (*McPhee, 2e, p 65.*) *Mycoplasma pneumoniae* shows no more predilection for HIV and AIDS patients than it does for persons with intact immune systems. *Pneumocystis carinii* pneumonia occurs almost exclusively in persons with HIV and AIDS and not in persons with intact immune systems, usually when the CD4 lymphocyte count falls below about 450 cells/μL. However, prophylaxis with trimethoprim-sulfamethoxazole or pentamidine aerosols now prevents most of the cases of PCP. *Mycobacterium tuberculosis* occurs at a high rate in persons with AIDS; they can become infected and spread drug-resistant strains of *Mycobacterium tuberculosis* that are very difficult to treat especially if they exhibit resistance to both isoniazid and rifampin. *S. pneumoniae* and *H. influenzae* occur at high rates in persons with HIV and AIDS.

142. The answer is e. (*McPhee, 2e, p 65.*) *Mycobacterium tuberculosis* is an airborne microorganism that is deposited directly into the lower airways. The large microorganisms are caught in the nose and pharynx and colonize these structures, and the smaller microorganisms are deposited on the mucociliary blanket of the respiratory tree.

143. The answer is b. (*McPhee, 2e, p 65.*) *Pneumocystis carinii*, a common cause pneumonia in persons with late stage HIV and AIDS, was the most common cause of pneumonia in this group of persons until prophylaxis either with trimethoprim-sulfamethoxazole or pentamidine aerosol became a routine feature of their care.

144. The answer is d. *(McPhee, 2e, p 65.)* Persons with acute and chronic alcoholism become infected with *Klebsiella pneumoniae,* most often by aspiration. *K. pneumoniae* pneumonia often localizes in the upper lobe, sometimes the minor fissures bows downward, reflecting the bogginess of the upper lobe involved with this infection.

145. The answer is c. *(McPhee, 2e, p 65.)* Psittacine birds transmit *Chlamydia psittaci* to humans who come in contact with them or keep them as pets. The pneumonia appears as an atypical pneumonia (patchy, interstitial infiltrate) on chest roentgenogram, similar to other atypical pneumonias such as *Mycoplasma pneumoniae* pneumonia. It also responds to treatment with a broad spectrum antibiotic, such as a macrolide or doxycycline.

146. The answer is e. *(McPhee, 2e, p 65.)* Persons suffering from chronic lung disease develop pneumonia due to *Moraxella catarrhalis,* and also to *S. pneumoniae* and *H. influenzae.* Very often, their sputum is colonized by one or more of the microorganisms that gains entrance to the lower respiratory tract because of damage to the respiratory tract cilia and the mucociliary blanket.

147. The answer is d. *(McPhee, 2e, p 67.)* Viruses account for 30 to 40% of the cases of infectious diarrhea in the U.S.; rotavirus is the predominant virus, especially in infants and children. The main bacterial pathogens are *Helicobacter pylori* and various *E. coli* serotypes. *Crytposporidium* causes a particularly severe diarrhea in persons with HIV and AIDS and a very low CD4 lymphocyte count, usually less than 100 cells/μL.

148. The answer is e. *(McPhee, 2e, p 68.)* On a worldwide basis, the single most important bacteria that causes diarrhea is *E. coli,* of which several main types play important roles in diarrhea illnesses. These include the following types: enteroaggregative, enteropathogenic, enterotoxigenic, enteroinvasive, and enterohemorrhagic. Enterotoxigenic occur more widely in acute diarrhea than the other types. They produce two enterotoxins that adversely affect the mucosal cells of the small intestine, resulting in a watery diarrhea. Enterohemorrhagic *E. coli* of serotype O157:H7 is associated with the severe hemolytic-uremia syndrome, as well as nonbloody diarrhea, noninflammatory diarrhea, and thrombotic thrombocytopenia purpura. It also produces toxins that are Shiga-like, called verotoxins, composed of one large protein unit (the A subunit) and five small subunits (the B subunit) that bind the toxin to the intestinal cell, stop intracellular protein synthesis, and eventually kill the intestinal cells.

149. The answer is c. *(Fauci, 14e, p 797.)* Certain bacteria can aggregate at the mucosal wall as a mechanism of producing diarrhea, but an antigen-antibody reaction is involved. Enterotoxin, cytotoxin, and invasion of the mucosal wall are mechanisms of bacterial diarrhea in differing bacterial pathogens. *Salmonella typhi* and *Yersinia enterocolitica* are two pathogens that penetrate mucosal wall, multiply in lymph nodes and Peyer's Patches, and then spread to the bloodstream, causing enteric fever. Characteristically, these two microorganisms cause destruction of mucosal cells, unlike the other pathogens of acute diarrhea.

150. The answer is e. *(Fauci, 14e, pp 767–776.)* The chemicals listed are mediators of sepsis, and additional mediators include platelet-activating factor, endothelium-derived relaxing factor, kinin, coagulation, and myocardial depressant substance. However, it is only nitric oxide, produced by inducible nitric oxide synthetase (iNOS), that has been shown to be the mediator of septic shock.

151. The answer is d. *(McPhee, 2e, p 44.)* CD4 T lymphocyte is the main CD antigen involved in HIV and AIDS. HIV infection destroys the CD4 lymphocytes. The CD8 lymphocytes increase in a reciprocal manner in HIV.

152. The answer is e. *(McPhee, 2e, p 44.)* Bone marrow stimulation is not involved; viral proteins show toxicity not only for the CD4 lymphocytes but also for the marrow, suppressing its function. Apoptosis (programmed cell death), autoimmune destruction of CD4 lymphocytes, and syncytium formation contribute to the decrease in CD4 lymphocytes.

153. The answer is d. *(McPhee, 2e, p 44.)* Usually, HIV progresses slowly, and the beginning of immunosuppression is about 5 to 10 years after the onset of infection. Infection begins with an acute, brief, febrile viral syndrome, followed by a long symptom-free period until the CD4 T lymphocyte begins to decline, providing evidence of immunosuppression.

154. The answer is b. *(McPhee, 2e, pp 45–48.)* *Pneumocystis carinii* pneumonia is a common complication of HIV and AIDS, and it is the most common opportunistic infection in HIV and AIDS. It can be prevented in most persons by prophylaxis with trimethoprim-sulfamethoxazole or pentamidine aerosols. A serious lung infection, it can be life threatening. All persons with HIV and AIDS experience one or more of the complications discussed in questions 170 to 177, especially as their immune system progressively fails.

155. The answer is a. *(McPhee, 2e, pp 45–48.)* *Candida albicans* causes thrush of the mouth and a severe esophagitis characterized by severe pain and dysphagia.

156. The answer is e. *(McPhee, 2e, pp 45–48.)* Biliary tract disease of differing types can be caused by *Cryptosporidium,* a protozoa that infects the gastrointestinal tract in many patients with HIV and AIDS.

157. The answer is d. *(McPhee, 2e, pp 45–48.)* Herpesvirus infections are common in persons with HIV and AIDS. Many of them experience reactivation of latent *Herpesvirus varicellae* infections or shingles that are very painful. Until the lesions crust over, they potentially can communicate chickenpox to susceptible persons.

158. The answer is e. *(McPhee, 2e, pp 45–48.)* Toxoplasmosis, acquired from infected cats, causes space occupying lesions, accompanied by central nervous system symptoms.

159. The answer is a. *(McPhee, 2e, pp 45–48.)* Kaposi's sarcoma typically causes purplish, dense, localized skin lesions of varying size and also visceral organ involvement. The lesions progress slowly but can become large and fulminant. Kaposi's sarcoma in AIDS occurs mainly in homosexual men.

160. The answer is b. *(McPhee, 2e, pp 45–48.)* Cytomegalovirus, also a herpesvirus, causes retinitis that leads progressively to complete blindness without treatment.

161. The answer is d. *(McPhee, 2e, pp 45–48.)* Wasting and cachexia are caused by a bloodstream infection with *Mycobacterium avium* complex (MAN), which includes *M. avium* and *M. intracellulare.* MAN organisms occur widely in nature—soil and animals—and spread to humans. However, almost only immunosuppressed persons become infected, especially persons with AIDS who possess few CD4 lymphocytes.

162. The answer is d. *(Fauci, 14e, pp 1051–1052.)* Infection with *Coxiella burnetii* (or Q fever) represents an occupational hazard of veterinarians. Q fever is characterized by fever, extreme fatigue, and headache, and about one-fourth of persons with the infection develop thrombocytopenia, unlike in the other infections. *Mycoplasma pneumoniae* infection is insidious and causes pneumonia as does *Chlamydia pneumoniae* infection; thrombocytopenia is not a characteristic of these infections. Influenza develops rapidly, in 2 to 3 days from exposure.

163. The answer is a. *(Fauci, 14e, p 1445.)* Pneumococcal polysaccharide vaccine is composed of purified polysaccharides from 23 serotypes of the pneumococcus that account for about 90% of infections. The polysaccharides are purified from the capsule of the organism grown in broth. The formulation remains unchanged from introduction of the vaccine in 1983. By comparison, the components of the influenza vaccine, the only other vaccine for prevention of respiratory tract disease, change annually because of antigenic drift and shift that occurs in the virus in nature. Additionally, a second pneumococcal vaccine was licensed recently for use in children under 2 years of age composed of 7 polysaccharides conjugated to a protein carrier to provide a superior antibody response in this age group compared with the 23-valent vaccine.

164. The answer is c. *(Fauci, 14e, p 1053.)* *Mycoplasma pneumoniae* pneumonia occurs predominantly in adolescents and young adults and also in elderly adults. It begins insidiously with fever, cough, and scant white sputum, but not hemoptysis. The cold agglutinin antibodies are elevated in this infection, usually in about one-half of cases and not in the other infections. The chest x-ray is usually positive and the infiltrate is interstitial, mainly in the lower lobe on one side; occasionally, it involves both lungs.

165. The answer is d. *(Fauci, 14e, pp 1176–1177.)* In *E. histolytica* clinical infection, antibody is not protective, and titers correlate with the duration of illness and not the severity. Clinical infection fails to induce immunity to recurrent colonization. Episodes of recurrent colitis are unusual nonetheless.

166. The answer is d. *(Fauci, 14e, pp 1120–1121.)* Because of the real, but very small, risk of paralysis associated with the administration of live oral poliovirus (OPV) vaccine, especially in adults, inactivated poliovirus vaccine (IPV) is now the recommended vaccine for use in children and adults.

167. The answer is d. *(Fauci, 14e, p 1013.)* Adults younger than 35 years of age with PPD skin test reactivity (meaning induration, not redness) of 10-mm diameter or more and at risk of tuberculosis should be given INH prophylaxis for 6 months. HIV-infected adults with PPD induration of 5 mm or more should be given INH prophylaxis. INH prophylaxis is not recommended for persons in the other three groups listed.

168. The answer is d. *(Fauci, 14e, pp 785–786; 832.)* Injection drug abusers usually contaminate their bloodstream from the skin. However, much less commonly than skin, contaminated drug serves as the source of the pathogen. The other organ systems do not serve as a source of the pathogens of endocarditis in drug abusers.

169. The answer is d. *(Fauci, 14e, p 1094.)* Isolation of virus from blood or demonstration of a fourfold or greater rise in antibody is the most reliable means of diagnosis of an acute infection of CMV. Excretion of CMV in the urine or the saliva can persist for months. Clinical findings alone are insufficient to differentiate CMV infection from other acute virus infections.

170. The answer is b. (*Fauci, 14e, p 1094.*) The anemia that develops in severe infections of falciparum malaria results from accelerated erythrocyte destruction and removal by the spleen. Few patients show significant bleeding with disseminated intravascular coagulation. Lactic acidosis occurs in severe malaria in part due to lactate production by the parasites. Increased Kuppfer cells in the liver and inadequate iron storage do not account for the anemia.

171. The answer is c. (*Fauci, 14e, p 985.*) About 60% of cases occur in children and do not cause fever in most cases, but patients usually develop systemic systems including weight loss, anorexia, and fatigue. Painful regional lymphadenopathy persists for weeks, and occasionally the involved nodes can become suppurative. However, cultures of lymph nodes or other tissues are rarely positive. Cat-scratch disease uncomplicated by central nervous sytem disease is a self-limiting disease of several weeks or months.

172. The answer is c. (*Fauci, 14e, p 985.*) The rash is impetigo, which is caused by group A streptococci, occasionally by other streptococci, and also by *Staphylococcus aureus*. It occurs in children who have poor hygiene, and the streptococci, which colonize the skin, gain entrance through a break in the skin, such as a scratch or an insect bite. The rash is painless, unlike herpes simplex or shingles, which is due to *Herpesvirus varicellae*. Herpes simplex occurs on the face and mouth and genitals; shingles follows the distribution of a nerve, mainly the temporal nerve and the intracostal nerves. Scarlet fever, also due to streptococci, characteristically covers the trunk and extremities with a fine papular rash, sparing the palms and soles. Erysipelas is a streptococcal cellulitis.

Cardiovascular

Questions

DIRECTIONS: Each item below contains a question or incomplete statement followed by suggested responses. Select the **one best** response to each question.

173. Which one of the following ECG components varies with heart rate?

a. PR interval
b. QRS duration
c. ST segment
d. QT interval
e. QRS voltage

174. Which of the following cardiac parameters decreases during pregnancy?

a. Cardiac output
b. Stroke volume
c. Heart rate
d. Blood volume
e. Systemic vascular resistance

175. Which of the following occurs during systole?

a. Blood passes from atria into the ventricles
b. The atrioventricular (AV) valves are open
c. Rapid ventricular filling occurs
d. The ventricles contract
e. Atrial contraction propels final proportion of blood into ventricles

176. Cardiac output, the volume of blood ejected from the ventricles in 1 minute, is equal to which of the following?

a. The product of heart rate and stroke volume
b. The product of contractility and preload
c. The difference between preload and afterload
d. The product of heart rate and preload
e. The difference between contractility and afterload

Review the Frank-Starling curve to answer questions 177–179.

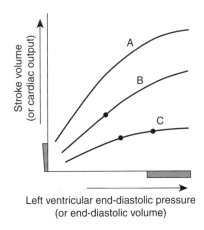

Left ventricular end-diastolic pressure
(or end-diastolic volume)

177. Curve A corresponds to which of the following?

a. A patient in congestive heart failure
b. A patient with normal left ventricular function who is receiving intravenous dobutamine as part of a diagnostic study for ischemia
c. A patient in congestive heart failure due to diastolic dysfunction
d. A normal person whose stroke volume increases as preload increases
e. A patient with congestive heart failure treated with a positive inotrope

178. Curve B corresponds to which of the following?

a. A patient in congestive heart failure treated with a positive inotrope
b. A patient in congestive heart failure due to systolic function
c. A normal person whose stroke volume increases as preload increases
d. A patient with normal left ventricular function who is receiving intravenous dobutamine as part of a diagnostic study for ischemia
e. A patient in congestive heart failure due to diastolic dysfunction

179. Curve C corresponds to which of the following?

a. A patient in congestive heart failure due to systolic dysfunction
b. A normal person whose stroke volume increases as preload increases
c. A patient with normal left ventricular function who is receiving intravenous dobutamine as part of a diagnostic study for ischemia
d. A patient in congestive heart failure due to diastolic function
e. A patient in congestive heart failure treated with a positive inotrope

Review the left ventricular pressure volume loop to answer questions 180–183.

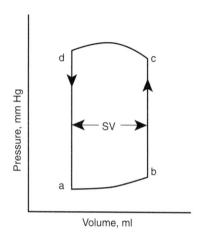

180. Which of the following represent the mitral valve opening?
a. Point A
b. Line A–B
c. Point B
d. Line B–C
e. Point C

181. Which of the following represent the mitral valve closing?
a. Line A–B
b. Point B
c. Point C
d. Line B–C
e. Point D

182. Which of the following represent the aortic valve opening?
a. Point A
b. Line B–C
c. Point C
d. Line C–D
e. Point D

183. Which of the following represent left ventricular ejection?

a. Point A
b. Point B
c. Line B–C
d. Line C–D
e. Point C

Review the diagram of an ECG tracing for questions 184–187.

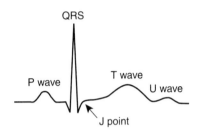

184. Which of the following would represent left or right atrial enlargement on a surface electrocardiogram?

a. Wide or tall P wave
b. Wide or tall T wave
c. A prominent U wave
d. An elevated J point
e. A large QRS voltage

185. Which of the following is often noted during hypokalemia?

a. Prominent P wave
b. Prominent QRS complex
c. Long Q–T interval
d. Prominent U wave
e. J point elevation

186. Which of the following represent repolarization of the ventricles?

a. P wave
b. QRS complex
c. T wave
d. J point
e. U wave

187. Which of the following would widen if a bundle branch block were present?

a. P wave
b. QRS complex
c. T wave
d. J point
e. U wave

188. A normal frontal plane QRS axis is

a. +90° to +180°
b. −30° to −90°
c. −30° to +90°
d. 0° to +150°
e. 0° to +90°

189. Which of the following associations is correct?

a. Hypokalemia: shortened Q–T interval
b. Hypercalcemia: long Q–T interval
c. Hypercalcemia: flattened T waves
d. Hypocalcemia: U waves
e. Hyperkalemia: peaked T waves

Review the diagram of electrolyte flux and the phase of the action potential for questions 190–194.

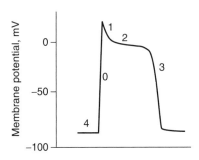

190. Influx of sodium ions

a. Phase 0
b. Phase 1
c. Phase 2
d. Phase 3
e. Phase 4

191. May involve chloride ion movement

a. Phase 0
b. Phase 1
c. Phase 2
d. Phase 3
e. Phase 4

192. Resting state

a. Phase 0
b. Phase 1
c. Phase 2
d. Phase 3
e. Phase 4

193. Mediated via slow conduction channels

a. Phase 0
b. Phase 1
c. Phase 2
d. Phase 3
e. Phase 4

194. Rapid potassium exit

a. Phase 0
b. Phase 1
c. Phase 2
d. Phase 3
e. Phase 4

195. Which of the following arterial pulse waveforms is consistent with severe left ventricular impairment?

a. Parvus et tardus pulse
b. Bisferiens pulse
c. Pulsus alternans
d. Hyperkinetic pulse
e. Dicrotic pulse

196. Which of the following arteriole pulse waveforms is consistent with aortic stenosis?

a. Pulsus alternans
b. Pulsus tardus
c. Bisferiens pulse
d. Dicrotic pulse
e. Parvus et tardus pulse

197. Which of the following conditions is consistent with a hypokinetic arterial pulse?

a. Left ventricular failure
b. Hypovolemia
c. Restrictive pericardial disease
d. Mitral stenosis
e. All of these

198. Which of the following statements is true of a reversed splitting of the first heart sound?

a. The mitral component follows the tricuspid component
b. It may be present in severe mitral stenosis
c. It may be present with a left atrial myxoma
d. It may be present with a left bundle branch block
e. All of these

Items 199–204

Match the following heart sounds with the appropriate description:

199. Which of the following heart sounds is produced by closure of the AV valves?

a. S3
b. Opening snap
c. S1
d. S2
e. S4

200. Which of the following heart sounds is produced by closure of the semilunar (aortic and pulmonic) valves?

a. S3
b. Opening snap
c. S1
d. S2
e. S4

201. Which of the following heart sounds is low pitched and produced in the ventricle at the termination of rapid filling, heard in normal children and in patients with increased cardiac output?

a. S3
b. Opening snap
c. S1
d. S2
e. S4

202. Which of the following heart sounds is low pitched, presystolic sound of ventricular filling produced by atrial contraction?

a. S1
b. Opening snap
c. Midsystolic click
d. S3
e. S4

203. Which of the following heart sounds is high pitched, early diastolic sound, usually due to mitral stenosis?

a. S1
b. Opening snap
c. Midsystolic click
d. S3
e. S4

204. Which of the following heart sounds is often caused by mitral or tricuspid valve prolapse?

a. S1
b. Opening snap
c. Midsystolic click
d. S3
e. S4

205. The onset of the QRS complex on surface ECG corresponds to which action potential phase?

a. Phase I
b. Phase II
c. Phase III
d. Phase IV
e. Phase 0

206. The isoelectric ST segment on surface ECG corresponds to which action potential phase?

a. Phase I
b. Phase II
c. Phase III
d. Phase IV
e. Phase 0

207. The T wave on the surface ECG corresponds to which action potential phase?

a. Phase I
b. Phase II
c. Phase III
d. Phase IV
e. Phase 0

208. Which of the following is represented by a prolonged PR interval and is due to delayed AV conduction?

a. Asystole
b. Third-degree AV block type
c. Second-degree AV block type I
d. First-degree AV block
e. Second-degree AV block type II

209. Which of the following AV blocks is characterized by progressive PR interval prolongation prior to loss of AV conduction?

a. First-degree AV block
b. Second-degree AV block type I
c. Second-degree AV block type II
d. Third-degree AV block

210. Which of the following is the correct sequence for myocardial depolarization?

a. AV node →
    bundle of His →
    atria
b. Bundle of His →
    AV node →
    left ventricle →
c. Sinoatrial (SA node) →
    AV node →
    bundle of His →
    right and left ventricles
d. SA node →
    left ventricle →
    bundle of His

211. Which ECG leads represent the inferior cardiac wall?

a. V_1, V_2
b. V_3, V_4
c. aVR
d. I, aVL
e. II, III, aVF

212. Which of the following produces a diastolic murmur?

a. Aortic regurgitation
b. Aortic stenosis
c. Mitral regurgitation
d. Supravalvular aortic stenosis
e. Tricuspid regurgitation

213. Loss of P waves on surface ECG is consistent with

a. First-degree AV block
b. Atrial flutter
c. Atrial fibrillation
d. Sinus bradycardia
e. Second-degree AV block type I

214. The arrow indicates

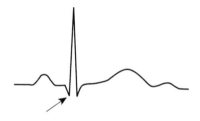

a. R wave
b. S wave
c. QS wave
d. Q wave
e. T wave

215. Cardiac output is the product of

a. Preload × stroke volume
b. Afterload × heart rate
c. Heart rate × stroke volume
d. Contractility × preload
e. Preload × heart rate

216. Which of the following is true regarding right ventricular hypertrophy?

a. The hypertrophy may result from aortic valve stenosis
b. The hypertrophy is characterized by poor R wave progression in leads V_1 to V_3
c. The hypertrophy is usually associated with left axis deviation
d. There are no associated ST-T wave changes
e. The hypertrophy is secondary to an atrial septal defect

Cardiovascular

Answers

173. The answer is d. *(Fauci, 14/e, p 1238.)* The standard surface ECG is divided into various intervals and segments. The small horizontal "boxes" on a standard ECG each equal 0.04 s, five small "boxes" comprise one large box, measuring 0.20 s. The P wave represents atrial depolarization. The PR interval is measured from the beginning of the P wave to the beginning of the QRS complex and represents AV conduction. A normal PR interval measurement is 0.12 to 0.20 s. A PR interval greater than 0.20 s is referred to as a first-degree AV block. The QRS complex on a standard surface ECG represents ventricular depolarization. Normal QRS duration is less than 0.10 s. If the QRS duration is greater than 0.10 s, a bundle branch block is most likely present. The ST segment is the most usual site evaluated for the presence of ischemia or injury. The ST segment is elevated in acute myocardial injury and depressed in the presence of myocardial ischemia. The QT interval varies with heart rate. This interval represents both ventricular

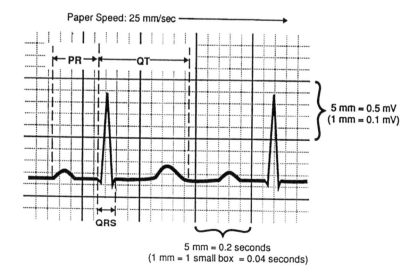

Paper Speed: 25 mm/sec

5 mm = 0.5 mV
(1 mm = 0.1 mV)

5 mm = 0.2 seconds
(1 mm = 1 small box = 0.04 seconds)

depolarization and repolarization. The QT interval increases with brady-cardia and decreases as the heart rate increases. The normal QT interval depends on heart rate, but a corrected "QT interval" may be calculated as the QT interval divided by the square root of the R–R interval. The normal corrected QT interval is less than 0.44 s. Prolongation of the QT interval is clinically important, because it can lead to fatal dysrhythmias such as tor-sades de pointes.

174. The answer is e. *(Fauci, 14/e, p 26.)* Normal cardiovascular changes that occur with pregnancy include decreased systemic vascular resistance, increased blood volume, increased stroke volume, increased heart rate, and increased cardiac output. These changes are quite well tolerated during normal pregnancy but, with preexisting cardiac disease, these changes may not be well tolerated. Because of these normal car-diovascular changes during pregnancy, new systolic murmurs may develop, as well as the presence of a third heart sound. In a physiologi-cally normal heart, these developments are considered normal during pregnancy.

175. The answer is d. *(Lilly, pp 18–19.)* The cardiac cycle consists of both systole and diastole. During diastole, the AV valves are open and the atrial and ventricular pressures are essentially equal. Left atrial contraction occurs in late diastole, causing a small increase in pressure in the left atrium and left ventricle. Left ventricular systole initiates left ventricular contraction. The mitral valve closes as left ventricular pressure overcomes left atrial pressure; this represents the mitral component of the first heart sound. As left ventricular pressure continues to increase, the aortic valve opens and blood is ejected. As the ventricles then begin to relax, the pul-monic and aortic valves close, causing the second heart sound. As left ventricular pressure continues to drop, the aortic valve opens. The con-traction of both ventricles initiates systole and does not occur during dia-stole.

176. The answer is a. *(Lilly, pp 148–150.)* Cardiac output, which is the volume of blood ejected from the ventricle in 1 min, changes regularly as the body's needs change and is the product of stroke volume and heart rate.

Therefore, for instance, when an individual begins to exercise and heart rate increases, the cardiac output will increase as well. Stroke volume is merely the volume of blood ejected from the ventricle during systole. Preload is the ventricular wall tension present at the end of diastole. Afterload is the ventricular wall tension present during contraction and is a function of aortic pressure and volume and thickness of the ventricular cavity. Contractility is actual measurement of the strength of contractile force. Contractility and preload contribute positively to stroke volume, whereas increased afterload decreases stroke volume. Thus, ultimately contractility, preload, afterload, stroke volume, and heart rate are all contributors to cardiac output.

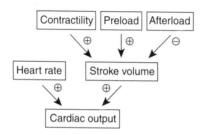

177–179. The answers are 177: b; 178: c; 179: a. *(Lilly, p 150.)* Frank-Starling curves or ventricular function curves are diagrams that show the relationship between stroke volume or cardiac output and preload or left ventricular end-diastolic volume. In normal individuals, as left ventricular end-diastolic pressure or preload increases, stroke volume will increase proportionately. In patients who suffer heart failure, increased left ventricular end-diastolic pressure is not met with increased stroke volume, because the contractility is depressed and is unable to function; thus, the patient ultimately experiences heart failure. If an individual with normal contractility is administered a positive inotropic agent, such as dobutamine, the contractility will increase without a necessary increase in preload. This is reflected by curve (A) on the Frank-Starling curve. The middle curve (B) represents a normal individual whose stroke volume will increase as preload increases. The bottom curve (C) represents a patient with congestive heart failure in that increasing this individual's preload will not be met with an increase in stroke volume and will result in pulmonary edema.

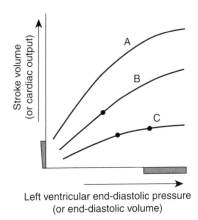

Left ventricular end-diastolic pressure
(or end-diastolic volume)

180–183. The answers are 180: a; 181: b; 182: c; 183: d. *(Lilly, p 151.)* A normal left ventricular volume loop is represented here. The mitral valve opens at point A. Diastolic filling ensues, represented by the line A–B, at which point ventricular contraction begins and the mitral valve closes at point B. Isometric contraction (the aortic valve is not yet open) is represented by the line B–C, indicating the increase in pressure in the left ventricle. As the left ventricular pressure maximizes, the aortic valve opens at point C. Line C–D thus corresponds with left ventricular ejection, and the aortic valve closes at point D. Line D–A thus represents isometric relaxation and subsequent reopening of the mitral valve at point A.

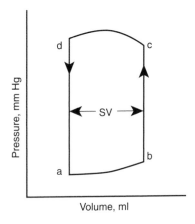

184. The answer is a. *(Fauci, 14/e, pp 1238–1242.)* The waveforms on a standard surface ECG include the P wave, which precedes the QRS complex. It is usually a rather small upward deflection that represents atrial depolarization. Thus, if right or left atrial enlargement were present, the P wave would reflect these changes. During right atrial enlargement, the P wave is tall, as seen in lead II. During left atrial enlargement, the P wave tends to become widened and biphasic, which is best seen in leads V_1 and V_2. Electrolyte abnormalities are common causes of changes on surface ECG. Hypokalemia results in the presence of U waves, which is a relatively low-devoltage deflection after the T wave. U waves are nonspecific and may be present for other reasons, but they are a classic finding in hypokalemia. The QRS complex is usually the largest complex on the surface tracing. This complex represents depolarization of the left and right ventricles. Normal QRS duration is less than 0.1 s. If a right or left His bundle is blocked, this results in a widened QRS complex representing abnormal ventricular depolarization. The third waveform on a standard surface ECG is the T wave, which represents repolarization of the ventricles. The T wave may show changes during myocardial ischemia, as well as electrolyte abnormalities, and may be altered by many pharmacologic agents.

185. The answer is d. *(Fauci, 14/e, pp 1238–1242.)* The waveforms on a standard surface ECG include the P wave, which precedes the QRS complex. It is usually a rather small upward deflection that represents atrial depolarization. Thus, if right or left atrial enlargement were present, the P wave would reflect these changes. During right atrial enlargement, the P wave is tall, as seen in lead II. During left atrial enlargement, the P wave tends to become widened and biphasic, which is best seen in leads V_1 and V_2. Electrolyte abnormalities are common causes of changes on the surface of an ECG. Hypokalemia results in the presence of U waves, which is a relatively low-devoltage deflection after the T wave. U waves are nonspecific and may be present for other reasons, but they are a classic finding in hypokalemia. The QRS complex is usually the largest complex on the surface tracing. This complex represents depolarization of the left and right ventricles. Normal QRS duration is less than 0.1 s. If a right or left His bundle is blocked, this results in a widened QRS complex representing abnormal ventricular depolarization. The third waveform on a standard surface ECG is the T wave, which represents repolarization of the ventricles. The T wave may show changes during myocardial ischemia, as well as electrolyte abnormalities, and may be altered by many pharmacologic agents.

186. The answer is c. (*Fauci, 14/e, pp 1238–1242.*) The waveforms on a standard surface ECG include the P wave, which precedes the QRS complex. It is usually a rather small upward deflection that represents atrial depolarization. Thus, if right or left atrial enlargement were present, the P wave would reflect these changes. During right atrial enlargement, the P wave is tall, as seen in lead II. During left atrial enlargement, the P wave tends to become widened and biphasic, which is best seen in leads V_1 and V_2. Electrolyte abnormalities are common causes of changes on the surface of an ECG. Hypokalemia results in the presence of U waves, which is a relatively low-devoltage deflection after the T wave. U waves are nonspecific and may be present for other reasons, but they are a classic finding in hypokalemia. The QRS complex is usually the largest complex on the surface tracing. This complex represents depolarization of the left and right ventricles. Normal QRS duration is less than 0.1 s. If a right or left His bundle is blocked, this results in a widened QRS complex representing abnormal ventricular depolarization. The third waveform on a standard surface ECG is the T wave, which represents repolarization of the ventricles. The T wave may show changes during myocardial ischemia, as well as electrolyte abnormalities, and may be altered by many pharmacologic agents.

187. The answer is b. (*Fauci, 14/e, pp 1238–1242.*) The waveforms on a standard surface ECG include the P wave, which precedes the QRS complex. It is usually a rather small upward deflection that represents atrial depolarization. Thus, if right or left atrial enlargement were present, the P wave would reflect these changes. During right atrial enlargement, the P wave is tall, as seen in lead II. During left atrial enlargement, the P wave tends to become widened and biphasic, which is best seen in leads V_1 and V_2. Electrolyte abnormalities are common causes of changes on the surface of an ECG. Hypokalemia results in the presence of U waves, which is a relatively low-devoltage deflection after the T wave. U waves are nonspecific and may be present for other reasons, but they are a classic finding in hypokalemia. The QRS complex is usually the largest complex on the surface tracing. This complex represents depolarization of the left and right ventricles. Normal QRS duration is less than 0.1 s. If a right or left His bundle is blocked, this results in a widened QRS complex representing abnormal ventricular depolarization. The third waveform on a standard surface ECG is the T wave, which represents repolarization of the ventricles. The T wave may show changes during myocardial ischemia, as well as electrolyte abnormalities, and may be altered by many pharmacologic agents.

188. The answer is c. *(Lilly, pp 57–67.)* The standard surface ECG is recorded from 12 leads. Leads V_1 through V_6 are placed on the anterior chest and are referred to as the chest leads. Leads aVR, aVF, and aVL are unipolar limb leads and are averaged together to create a standard reference. The aVR selects the right arm as the positive electrode, the aVF selects the left leg as the positive electrode, and the aVL selects the left arm as the positive electrode. Leads I, II, and III are also limb leads but are bipolar. Lead I designates the left arm as the positive electrode and the right arm as negative. Lead II has the left leg designated as the positive electrode and the right arm as the negative electrode. Lead III has the left arm designated as the negative electrode and the left leg as the positive electrode. When the six limb leads are interposed, a reference system is devised. The main QRS electrical axis may be determined by averaging the forces created during ventricular depolarization. The normal frontal plane QRS axis is −30 to approximately +90. An axis more negative than −30° indicates left axis deviation, and an axis greater than +90° indicates right axis deviation. The axis is determined by the positive or negative direction of the QRS complex in each of the limb leads.

189. The answer is e. *(Lilly, p 79.)* Electrolyte abnormalities affect various portions of the surface ECG. Both hypercalcemia and hypocalcemia affect ventricular repolarization and are thus represented by changes in the QT interval. Hypercalcemia results in a shortened QT interval, whereas hypocalcemia results in a prolonged QT interval. Calcium does not affect the T wave; it specifically changes the ST portion of the QT interval. Hyperkalemia may be represented by very tall peaked T waves as potassium affects ventricular repolarization. Hypokalemia may be represented by U waves, which are small deflections following the T wave.

190–194. The answers are 190: a; 191: b; 192: e; 193: c; 194: d. *(Lilly, p. 12.)* Myocardial contraction ultimately results from electrical impulses. An action potential is created by ion fluxes through certain channels in the cellular membranes. Various cardiac cells are capable of electrical activity including the pacemaker cells of the SA and AV nodes, the Purkinje fibers, and the cardiac muscle cells. The action potential consists of phases I to IV and of phase 0. Phase 0 is caused by the rapid influx of sodium ions. This is the rapid depolarization phase of the action potential. Phase I is not well understood but is the first stage of repolarization. This phase is thought to include chloride ion movement. Phase II is controlled by the slow calcium channels and is commonly referred to as the plateau. The slow calcium influx is an important factor in myocyte contraction. Phase III consists largely of the exiting of potassium and returning of the resting potential to approximately −90 mV. Phase IV is simply the resting state prior to stimulation.

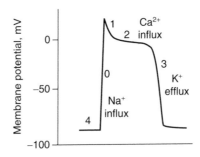

195–197. The answers are 195: c; 196: b; 197: e. (*Fauci, 14/e, p 1232.*) The arterial pulse may be palpitated in the periphery, or evaluation of the carotid may occur. Certain changes in the arterial pressure pulse occur with various pathologic conditions. Pulsus parvus, defined as a small weak pulse, is present when left ventricular stroke volume is decreased. A hypokinetic or weak pulse is commonly present due to conditions such as hypovolemia, heart failure, restrictive pericardial disease, or mitral stenosis. In pulsus tardus (late pulse) the systolic peak is delayed. It is common in aortic stenosis, because the left ventricular ejection is impeded because of the stenotic valve. A bisferiens pulse has two peaks and is common with aortic regurgitation. Pulsus alternans is a unique pattern during which the amplitude of the pulse changes or alternates in size with a stable heart rhythm. This is common in severe left ventricular dysfunction. In summary, examination of the arterial pressure pulse may lead to clues of existing pathology.

198. The answer is e. *(Fauci, 14/e, p 1234.)* The first heart sound consists of a mitral and tricuspid component. Normally, the mitral valve closes first, thus contributing to the first component of S_1. When there is reverse splitting of S_1, the mitral component follows the tricuspid component. This finding may be present in severe mitral stenosis and may be due to the presence of a left atrial myxoma, which often mimics mitral stenosis. Splitting may be present also with a left bundle branch block.

199–204. The answers are 199: c; 200: d; 201: a; 202: e; 203: b; 204: c. *(Fauci, 14/e, pp 1234–1235.)* The first heart sound is produced by closure of the mitral and tricuspid valves (the AV or atrioventricular valves). Normally, the mitral valve closure precedes the tricuspid valve closure; thus, the mitral valve contributes to the first component of S_1. The second heart sound is caused by the aortic and pulmonic valve closure. The aortic component is generally louder than the pulmonic component. The fixed splitting of the second heart sound is caused by atrial septal defect. Normally, the splitting of S_2 representing the difference in closure between the aortic and pulmonic valves varies with respiration. If an atrial septal defect is present, this variation does not occur, and the two components of S_2 are "fixed." A third heart sound is present in individuals with increased cardiac output. It is a low-pitched sound produced in the ventricle. In adults, this is a pathologic finding, but an S_3 is quite normal in young children. A fourth heart sound may be present and is produced by atrial contraction. The S_4 is a low-pitched sound produced during ventricular filling. It may be a normal finding in the elderly, because the left ventricle tends to "stiffen" with age. Obviously, because the sound is due to atrial contraction, it is absent in patients with atrial fibrillation. A classic finding of mitral stenosis is an opening snap that is a high-pitched early diastolic sound. An opening snap may be noted with tricuspid stenosis. Midsystolic clicks usually result from mitral or tricuspid prolapse and are due to unequal chordae tendineae.

205–207. The answers are 205: e; 206: b; 207: c. *(Fauci, 14/e, p 1238.)* The surface ECG tracing, which is a representation of the electrical activity of the heart, corresponds to the various phases of the ventricular action potential. The QRS complex on surface ECG represents ventricular depolarization. The intracellular activity during ventricular repolarization is a rapid influx of sodium and corresponds to phase 0 of the action potential. The isoelectric ST segment corresponds to continued ventricular depolarization and repolarization. This corresponds to the plateau phase or phase II. This phase is mediated via slow calcium channels. The T wave on surface ECG represents ventricular repolarization. Intracellularly, this corresponds to phase III, during which potassium rapidly exits the cells.

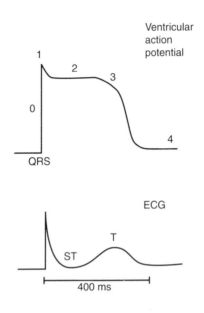

208. The answer is d.   (*Fauci, 14/e, p 1256.*) First-degree AV block is represented by a prolonged PR interval. This is due to delayed AV conduction. Second-degree AV block is divided into two types: I and II. Type I is an AV block above the level of the His bundle and is characterized by gradually prolonging PR intervals followed by a P wave that is not conducted to the ventricle. Second-degree AV block type II is generally due to disease of the His–Purkinje system. The PR interval does not gradually prolong, and there is sudden loss of a QRS complex following a P wave. Third-degree block is present when no AV conduction occurs. The atrium is depolarizing independently of the ventricle.

209. The answer is b.   (*Fauci, 14/e, p 1256.*) First-degree AV block is represented by a prolonged PR interval. This is due to delayed AV conduction.

Second-degree AV block is divided into two types: I and II. Type I is an AV block (Wenkebach heart block) above the level of the His bundle and is characterized by gradually prolonging PR intervals followed by a P wave that is not conducted to the ventricle. Second-degree AV block type II (classical heart block) is generally due to disease of the His–Purkinje system. The PR interval does not gradually prolong, and there is sudden loss of a QRS complex following a P wave. Third-degree block is present when no AV conduction occurs. The atrium is depolarizing independently of the ventricle.

210. The answer is c. *(Fauci, 14/e, pp 1237–1238.)* The SA node, which is the site of initiation of a depolarization that results in a normal heartbeat, consists of pacemaker cells that fire spontaneously. The impulse then proceeds to the conduction tissues in the AV node in the His bundle, both of which are in the AV junction. The bundle of His then divides into the right bundle and left bundle, and the impulse is then conducted to the right and left ventricular myocardium through the Purkinje fibers. The left bundle bifurcates into the left anterior fascicle and left posterior fascicle. The depolarization then continues through both ventricular walls, and ventricular contraction is triggered. Depolarization occurs from endocardium to epi-

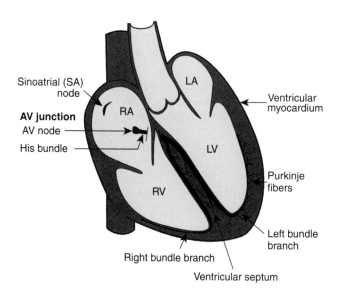

cardium. Thus, the correct sequence for myocardial depolarization is SA node through AV node through bundle of His and proceeding to both ventricles.

211. The answer is e. *(Lilly, p 76.)* The lead system on a standard surface ECG is designed so that certain leads represent specific segments of the left ventricle. The chest (or precordial) leads represent the anterior wall of the left ventricle with leads V_3 and V_4, the septal portion of the left ventricle with leads V_1 and V_2, and the low lateral portion of the left ventricle with leads V_5 and V_6. The high lateral wall is represented by the limb leads I and aVL. The inferior wall is represented by II, III, and aVF. Lead aVR does not represent a specific portion of the left ventricular muscle, because its positive electrode is the right arm.

212. The answer is a. *(Fauci, 14/e, p 1236.)* Systole is represented by left ventricular contraction and rapid ejection. Left ventricular systole must occur when the aortic valve is open. If the aortic valve is stenosed significantly, a systolic murmur will ensue as the blood flows through the constricted valve. If the mitral valve is incompetent or weakened during systole or left ventricular ejection, there will be backflow into the left atrium through the incompetent valve, and mitral regurgitation will result. As the backflow continues into the left atrium during systole, mitral regurgitation will result in a systolic murmur. Supravalvular aortic stenosis occurs when there is obstruction above the aortic valve structure proper and, again, the flow constriction will occur during ventricular systole, thus resulting in a systolic murmur. Tricuspid regurgitation, similar to mitral regurgitation, will also result in a systolic murmur due to backflow into the right atrium during right ventricular systole. In contrast, aortic regurgitation results in backflow into the left ventricle during relaxation. If the aortic valve is incompetent, as opposed to being stenosed, as the ventricle relaxes and the aortic valve is closed there will be regurgitation resulting in a diastolic murmur.

213. The answer is c. *(Lilly, p 71.)* Atrial depolarization is represented on the surface ECG as a P wave. Left or right atrial enlargement that exists is represented with increased voltage of the P wave. Atrial fibrillation occurs when there is chaotic, intermittently conducted atrial activity. Because there is no organized atrial contraction, no P wave is represented on the surface ECG.

214. The answer is d. *(Fauci, 14/e, p 1238.)* The QRS complex on a surface ECG represents ventricular depolarization. If the initial force of this complex is in a negative direction, this is referred to as a Q wave. The subsequent upward deflection is an R wave, and the final downward deflection is an S wave. A Q wave need not necessarily be present, if the initial force of the QRS complex is positive, then a Q wave by definition is not present. Pathologic Q waves occur when a myocardial infarction has occurred. Small Q waves are usually nonpathologic.

215. The answer is c. *(Lilly, pp 148–149.)* Cardiac output, which is defined as the volume of blood expelled from the ventricle per minute, is the product of heart rate and stroke volume. In turn, stroke volume (or the volume of blood that the ventricle ejects in systole) is determined by contractility, preload, and afterload.

216. The answer is e. *(Fauci, 14/e, p 1241.)* A cardiac hypertrophy of the various chambers is manifested on the surface ECG. If pulmonic valve stenosis is present, right ventricular pressure is significantly increased as the ventricle must contract against a stenotic valve. This results in hypertrophy of the right ventricle. The classic surface ECG findings include a prominent R wave in leads V_1 to V_3. Ventricular hypertrophy also often leads to ST depression and T wave changes in the precordial leads. This is often referred to as secondary repolarization changes or "strain pattern." If an atrial septal defect is present, the right ventricle is significantly volume overloaded, again resulting in right ventricular hypertrophy.

Pulmonary

Questions

DIRECTIONS: Each item below contains a question or incomplete statement followed by suggested responses. Select the **one best** response to each question.

217. Which one of the following hemodynamic findings is the main derangement of primary pulmonary hypertension?

a. Increased cardiac output early
b. Increased resistance to pulmonary blood flow
c. Decreased resistance to pulmonary blood flow
d. Decreased pulmonary capillary wedge pressure early
e. Normal diastolic filling of the left ventricle

218. Transudative pleural effusion is caused by which one of the following diseases?

a. Bacterial pneumonia
b. Malignancy
c. Cirrhosis
d. Sarcoidosis
e. Viral infection

219. When the exudative pleural effusion contains less than 60 mg/dL of glucose, which one of the following diseases is the most likely cause?

a. Eosophageal rupture
b. Cirrhosis
c. Malignant pleural effusion
d. Pancreatic pleural effusion
e. Diaphragmatic hernia

220. A 76-year-old man comes to your office in January with complaints of abrupt onset of cough, with small amounts of green sputum, worse in the morning, without any blood in it. He also has fever as high as 103°F, very rapid respirations (32/min), and chest pain on his right side, worsened with coughing. He exhibits some difficulty remembering the details of his illness. On the basis of these clinical findings, you consider a diagnosis of pneumonia. Which one choice would you make?

a. Obtain a chest x-ray and schedule him to return tomorrow
b. Treat his symptoms with antipyretics and cough syrup
c. Prescribe an oral antibiotic and also antipyretics and cough syrup and schedule him to return in 2 days
d. Admit him to the hospital in the intensive care unit for parenteral antibiotic treatment
e. Administer a tuberculin skin test (PPD), treat his symptoms with antipyretics and cough syrup, obtain a chest x-ray, and schedule him to return in 2 days for interpretation of the skin test

221. Which one of the following is true about silicosis?

a. Mesothelioma is a complication of silicosis
b. It is caused by exposure to asbestos fibers
c. An increased risk exists of developing tuberculosis in patients with silicosis
d. Silicosis generally presents as a pneumothorax on chest x-ray
e. Patients with silicosis should not receive any antituberculous therapy

222. Obstructive airway defect is characterized on pulmonary function testing by which one of the following?

a. Reduced FEV_1/FVC ratio
b. Decreased total lung capacity (TLC)
c. Reduced residual volume (RV)
d. Decreased residual volume/total lung capacity (RV/TLC)
e. Decrease in diffusing capacity (DLCO)

223. Which one of the following is the *first-line* therapy in the management of an *acute* asthma attack?

a. Steroids
b. β_2-agonists
c. Theophylline
d. Antibiotics
e. Magnesium sulfate

224. Which one of the following pathogens is a main cause of bronchiectasis?

a. Influenza virus
b. *Rhinovirus*
c. *Mycoplasma pneumoniae*
d. *Enterovirus*
e. Necrotizing fungal infections

225. The most frequent inherited disorder of hypercoagulability leading to pulmonary thromboembolism is

a. Deficiency in protein C
b. Deficiency in protein S
c. Deficiency in antithrombin III
d. Disorders of plasminogen
e. Activated protein C resistance (factor V Leiden)

226. ARDS is differentiated from acute lung injury (ALI) on the basis of which one of the following?

a. Presence of bilateral interstitial infiltrates on chest x-ray
b. Severity of hypoxemia with PaO_2/FiO_2 ratio of less than 200 mmHg
c. Increased pulmonary capillary wedge pressure
d. Reduced compliance
e. Systemic inflammatory response

227. Which one disease is the single most common indication for single lung transplantation?

a. Chronic obstructive pulmonary disease (COPD) either smoking induced or secondary to α-1-antitrypsin deficiency
b. Cystic fibrosis
c. Lung cancer
d. Idiopathic pulmonary fibrosis (IPF)
e. Primary pulmonary hypertension (PPH)

228. Which of the following statements is true about sarcoidosis?

a. The first manifestation is an accumulation of B lymphocytes
b. The giant cells in the granuloma lack inclusions
c. It is characterized by hypoglobulinemia
d. Sarcoid fails to clear spontaneously
e. It results from an exaggerated immune response

229. A 30-year-old male presents to the emergency room with shortness of breath and right-sided pleuritic chest pain. His chest x-ray in the emergency room is normal. An arterial blood gas is obtained while the patient is breathing room air. The results show a pH of 7.48, $PaCO_2$ of 35, PaO_2 of 68, and an oxygen saturation of 92%. What is his A-a gradient?

a. 20
b. 30
c. 40
d. 50
e. 60

230. Which one of the following eosinophilic pulmonary syndromes may present without any peripheral eosinophilia?

a. Loeffler's syndrome
b. Acute eosinophilic pneumonia
c. Chronic eosinophilic pneumonia
d. Allergic granulomatosis of Churg-Strauss
e. Hypereosinophilic syndrome

231. Exposure to asbestos fibers causes which one of the following x-ray findings?

a. Pulmonary vascular prominence
b. Pleural blebs
c. Enlarged right ventricle
d. Acute bronchopneumonia
e. Diffuse interstitial pulmonary fibrosis with irregular or linear opacities

232. In patients with COPD, long-term oxygen supplementation is prescribed if PaO_2 is

a. 55 mmHg or below
b. 65 mmHg
c. 70 mmHg
d. 75 mmHg
e. 80 mmHg or higher

233. The most common cause of mass in the posterior mediastinum is

a. Vascular
b. Esophageal diverticula
c. Neurogenic tumors
d. Lymphomas
e. Bronchogenic cysts

234. In obstructive sleep apnea (OSA) which one of the following contributes to the negative oropharyngeal pressure characteristic of OSA?

a. Pleural blebs
b. Laryngeal muscles hyperactivity
c. Occlusion of the upper airway at the level of the oropharynx
d. Low pharyngeal resistance
e. Low upstream (nasal) resistance

235. *Mycobacterium tuberculosis* is spread most effectively by which one of the following persons?

a. Persons whose sputum smear is negative for *Mycobacterium tuberculosis*, but whose culture is AFB-positive
b. Persons who are close contacts of tuberculosis patients
c. Persons recently infected who are culture-negative
d. Persons with proven extrapulmonary tuberculosis
e. Persons infected with *Mycobacterium tuberculosis* whose sputum smear is positive for AFB on microscopy

236. In which one of the following diseases would the occurrence of hemoptysis prompt a search for another disease as the cause of the hemoptysis?

a. Bronchogenic carcinoma
b. Acute bronchitis
c. Goodpasture's syndrome
d. Emphysema
e. Bronchiectasis

Pulmonary

Answers

217. The answer is b. *(Fauci, 14e, pp 1466–1468.)* The cardinal hemodynamic feature of primary pulmonary hypertension is increased resistance to blood flow. The pulmonary artery pressure becomes elevated, and in time, the cardiac output decreases, and late in the course, the pulmonary capillary wedge pressure increases because of impaired diastolic filling of the left ventricle.

218. Answer is c. *(Fauci, 14e, 1473.)* Transudative and exudative effusions can be distinguished by measuring the lactate dehydrogenase (LDH) and protein levels in the pleural fluid. Exudative effusions show a pleural fluid protein/serum protein greater than 0.5, pleural fluid LDH/serum LDH greater than 0.6, or pleural fluid LDH more than two-thirds normal upper limit for serum by these criteria. Only cirrhosis causes transudative effusions. Local factors contribute to exudative effusions in bacterial pneumonia, viral infections, malignancy, and sarcoidosis.

219. The answer is c. *(Fauci, 14e, pp 1473–1475.)* Exudative pleural effusions that contain less than 60 mg/DL of glucose are caused by malignancy, bacterial infections, and rheumatoid pleuritis. The other exudative effusions do not show low glucose levels. However, exudative effusions caused by esophageal rupture, pancreatic pleural effusion, and also malignancy show elevated amylase levels.

220. Answer is d. *(Fauci, 14e, 1441.)* Elderly patients and patients with other comorbid illnesses have a higher chance of complications following a community-acquired pneumonia, and they need to be admitted to the hospital for parenteral antibiotic treatment and close monitoring. Elderly patients with tachypnea and acute alteration in mental status are at high risk of adverse outcomes from pneumonia and need to treated in the hospital.

221. Answer is c. *(Fauci, 14e, p 1432.)* Workers exposed through sand blasting, tunneling through rock with high quartz content, or manufacture of abrasive soaps can develop silicosis. Chest x-ray findings include reticular pattern of irregular densities mostly in the upper lung zones. The nodular fibrosis may be progressive with formation of irregular masses of greater than 1 cm each. These masses can become quite large and coalesce to progressive massive fibrosis (PMF). Calcification of hilar lymph nodes may occur in as little as 20% of cases and can produce the characteristic "egg shell" calcification. Patients with silicosis are at greater risk of acquiring mycobacterium tuberculosis and atypical mycobacterial infections. Treatment or prophylaxis for tuberculosis is indicated in patients with silicosis and a positive tuberculin test.

222. The answer is a. *(Fauci, 14e, p 1412.)* Pulmonary function tests are divided into two subgroups: obstructive and restrictive defects. The hallmark of obstructive defect is a decrease in the expiratory flow rate, as manifested by a decrease in FEV_1/FVC ratio. Total lung capacity is normal or increased. Residual volume (RV) is elevated owing to the air trapping during expiration, which results in an increase of RV/TLC ratio. Vital capacity is frequently decreased in obstructive defects because of striking elevations in RV with only minor changes in TLC.

223. The answer is b. *(Fauci, 14e, p 1425.)* The most effective treatment for acute episodes of asthma is administration of aerosolized β_2-agonists. In emergency situations, they can be given every 20 min until the attack has subsided or the patient develops any side effects. Thereafter, the frequency can be reduced to every 2 to 4 h until the attack has totally subsided. Other drugs have some role in asthma but are not the first-line therapeutic agents for an acute attack.

224. The answer is a. *(Fauci, 14e; p 1446.)* Bronchiectasis is a consequence of inflammation and destruction of the bronchial walls. The main virus causes are influenza virus and adenovirus. *Rhinovirus, Mycoplasma pneumoniae,* and necrotizing fungal infections rarely cause bronchiectasis. Noninfectious causes include immune mediated inflammation, e.g., in allergic bronchopulmonary aspergillosis.

225. The answer is e. *(Fauci, 14e, p 1469.)* Activated protein C resistance is the single most common inherited predisposition to hypercoagulability. Its phenotype is associated with a single-point mutation, designated factor

V Leiden, which is more common than all other inherited hypercoagulable conditions combined. These include deficiencies in protein C, protein S, antithrombin III, and disorders of plasminogen.

226. The answer is b. *(Fauci, 14e, 1483.)* Acute respiratory distress syndrome (ARDS) and acute lung injury (ALI) are both characterized by bilateral interstitial infiltrates, normal pulmonary capillary wedge pressure, and low compliance. Both develop in response to infectious or systemic inflammatory conditions. However, the severity of hypoxemia, as defined by PaO_2/FiO_2 ratio, distinguishes the two syndromes from each other. In ARDS, patients have a refractory hypoxemia with a PaO_2/FiO_2 ratio of less than 200 mmHg, whereas in patients with ALI, this ratio is higher than 200.

227. The answer is a. *(Fauci, 14e, p 1491.)* COPD accounts for about 60% of all single lung transplants and about 30% of bilateral lung transplant. Cystic fibrosis accounts for approximately 36% of bilateral lung transplants and rests are miscellaneous reasons for lung transplant including idiopathic pulmonary fibrosis, primary pulmonary hypertension, and several other rarer lung diseases. Cancer in the lungs or outside the lungs would preclude patients from undergoing lung transplantation.

228. The answer is e. *(Fauci, 14e, 1922.)* Sarcoidosis is a chronic, multisystem disorder of unknown cause with an exaggerated immune response. It affects both sexes, although females seem to be slightly more susceptible than males. There is a remarkable diversity of the prevalence of sarcoidosis among certain ethnic and racial groups. The prevalence is from 10 to 40 per 100,000 in the U.S. In the U.S., most patients with sarcoidosis are black, with a ratio of blacks to whites ranging from 10:1 to 17:1. The therapy of choice for sarcoidosis is oral glucocorticoids. The disease responds well to steroids; however, the treatment for symptomatic sarcoid patients is administered usually over several months.

229. Answer is c. *(Fauci, 14e, p 1415.)* The patient most likely has a pulmonary embolism because of shortness of breath, right-sided pleuritic chest pain, a normal chest x-ray, and abnormal blood gases. A useful calculation is the assessment of Alveolar oxygenation and calculating the gradient between Alveolar and arterial partial pressures of the oxygen. At room air, the PaO_2 (Alveolar) can be calculated by the following formula. PaO_2 = $150 - 1.25 \times$ PaCO_2. Once PaO_2 is determined, the A-a gradient is simply the difference between PaO_2 and arterial PaO_2. In a healthy young person breathing room air, the PaO_2 − PaO_2 is normally less than 15 mmHg; this value increases with age and may be as high as 30 mmHg in elderly patients.

230. The answer is b. *(Fauci, 14e, p 1429.)* The group of idiopathic eosinophilic pneumonias consists of diseases of varying severity. Loeffler's syndrome was originally reported as migratory pulmonary infiltrates. In some patients, these may be secondary to parasites or drugs. Acute eosinophilic pneumonia is a recently described syndrome characterized by an acute febrile illness of less than 7 days in duration and may or may not present with peripheral eosinophilia. Chronic eosinophilic syndrome presents with significant systemic symptoms of weeks or months in duration and presents with peripheral eosinophilia. Allergic angiitis and granulomatosis of Churg-Strauss is a multisystem vasculitis that frequently involves skin, kidneys, and nervous system in addition to the lungs. This is also manifested by peripheral eosinophilia. The hypereosinophilic syndrome is characterized by the presence of more than 1500 eosinophils/μL of peripheral blood for 6 months or longer.

231. The answer is e. *(Fauci, 14e, p 1431.)* On x-ray examination, asbestos exposure causes diffuse interstitial pulmonary fibrosis that is slowly evolving and characterized by linear or irregular opacities of the lungs. Usually, about 10 years elapse since first exposure to asbestos and the development of asbestosis. Benign pleural effusions occur and these may resolve without treatment. However, pleural blebs, enlargement of the right ventricle, and increased prominence of the pulmonary vascular are not features of asbestosis on x-ray.

232. The answer is a. *(Fauci, 14e, p 1457.)* If PaO_2 is persistently below 55 mmHg, supplemental oxygen should be prescribed. However, if room air PaO_2 is between 55 and 60 mmHg, supplemental oxygen may still be prescribed if the patient has signs of cor pulmonale, secondary erythrocytosis, or signs of right heart failure. In patients with severe hypoxemia, supplemental oxygen improves exercise tolerance and neurophysiologic functions and alleviates pulmonary hypertension. It tends to improve survival if used greater than 15 to 19 h a day.

233. The answer is c. *(Fauci, 14e, p 1475.)* The most common tumor in the posterior mediastinum are the neurogenic tumors. Other masses found in the posterior mediastinum are meningoceles, gastroenteric cysts, and esophageal diverticula. The most common masses in the middle mediastinum are vascular masses, lymph node enlargement from metastases or granulomatous disease, and pleuropericardial and bronchogenic cysts. In the anterior mediastinum, the most common lesions are thymomas, lymphomas, teratomas, and thyroid masses.

234. Answer is c. *(Fauci, 14e, p 1480.)* Occlusion of the upper airway at the level of the oropharynx leading to negative oropharyngeal pressure represents the underlying mechanism in obstructive sleep apnea (OSA). Other contributing factors can be a small pharyngeal cavity, high pharyngeal compliance, and high upstream (nasal) resistance. Obesity contributes to OSA by increasing fat deposition in the soft tissues of the pharynx or by compressing the pharynx by superficial fat masses in the neck. In a few patients, structural compromise, such as adenotonsillar hypertrophy, retrognathia, or macroglossia, can contribute to the development of OSA also.

235. The answer is e. *(Fauci, 14e, p 1004–1005.)* *Mycobacterium tuberculosis* is most effectively spread by persons whose acid-fast bacilli (AFB) in their sputum is visible on microscopy, which means that the sputum contains about 100,000 organisms/mL or more. These persons usually have cavitary lung disease or endobronchial or laryngeal tuberculosis. Persons whose sputum smear is negative, but culture positive are much less infectious, and persons with extrapulmonary tuberculosis are not usually infectious.

236. The answer is d. *(Fauci, 14e, p 196–197.)* Hemoptysis is not a feature of emphysema. In patients with emphysema who present with hemoptysis, physicians must search for other causes. The most common cause of mild hemoptysis in the U.S. is acute bronchitis. Hemoptysis can occur because of a tracheobronchial source, pulmonary parenchymal source, primary vascular disease, coagulopathy, or immune mediated diseases, e.g., Goodpasture's syndrome.

Renal/Nephrology

Questions

DIRECTIONS: Each item below contains a question or incomplete statement followed by suggested responses. Select the **one best** response to each question.

237. Which is a common finding in acute glomerulonephritis?

a. Pulmonary congestion due to volume expansion
b. Hypovolemia due to tubular dysfunction
c. Uniformly progresses to chronic renal failure if untreated
d. Urine showing leukocytes and eosinophils

238. Which finding is fairly specific for chronic renal failure?

a. Anemia
b. Hyaline casts
c. Broad casts in urinalysis
d. Proteinuria
e. Hypocalcemia

239. Nephrotic syndrome is associated with

a. Excessive renal salt and water loss
b. Hyperlipidemia due to lipoprotein excess
c. Bleeding due to loss of clotting factors
d. Hypothyroidism due to loss of thyroid-binding globulin

240. A patient with chronic renal failure will be expected to have which of the following findings due to the mechanisms described?

a. Hypercalcemic due to elevated PTH hormone
b. Prolonged bleeding due to decreased synthesis of clotting factors
c. Anemia due to increased red cell destruction
d. Hypermagnesemia due to decreased renal excretion

241. A high fractional excretion of sodium is typically found in

a. Heart failure
b. Urinary tract obstruction
c. Acute tubular necrosis
d. Acute glomerulonephritis
e. Hepatorenal syndrome

242. Which of the following nephron segment is correctly paired with its function?

a. Distal tubule and bicarbonate reclamation
b. Loop of Henle and potassium regulation
c. Proximal tubule and urinary concentration
d. Collecting tubule and water regulation

243. Which of the following statements is true in the management of acute renal failure?

a. Metabolic acidosis is fully corrected with bicarbonate
b. Hyperphosphatemia is primarily managed with dialysis
c. Low-dose dopamine is used to shorten the duration of renal failure
d. Hypervolemia is managed with high-dose loop diuretics
e. Hyponatremia is corrected by administration of sodium salts

244. Which of the following describes bone abnormalities in patients with chronic renal failure?

a. Osteitis fibrosis cystica is a result of oversuppression of PTH
b. Adynamic bone disease is associated with myopathy
c. Osteomalacia is due to excessive accumulation of magnesium
d. Hyperparathyroidism responds well to 1,25 dihydroxyvitamin D
e. Amyloidosis is similar in etiology to patients who are not on dialysis

245. Which one of the following statements is true concerning hematologic disorders in CRF?

a. Resistance to erythropoietin is most commonly due to aluminum overload
b. Erythropoietin administration is associated with worsening hypertension
c. The major cause of death in CRF is sepsis
d. Abnormal bleeding responds best to platelet transfusion
e. Leukocyte function is generally unimpaired

246. Which of the following measures has not been shown to retard progression of renal failure?

a. Aggressive BP control
b. Decrease in protein intake
c. ACE inhibitors above other antihypertensives
d. Erythropoietin for anemia

247. In patients with chronic renal failure, which of the following adaptations are normal?

a. Fractional excretion of sodium increases due to suppression of aldosterone
b. Metabolic acidosis due to loss of bicarbonate in the urine
c. Increased potassium loss through extrarenal mechanisms
d. Decreased fractional excretion of water due to ADH resistance

248. Which of the following serologic finding is associated with linear staining of the glomerulus on immunofluorescence?

a. Anti-GBM antibody
b. Low complement immune complex glomerulonephritis
c. ANCA associated renal disease
d. Membranoproliferative glomerulonephritis

249. Antineutrophil cytoplasmic antibody (ANCA) is typically present in which systemic disease?

a. Goodpasture's syndrome
b. Wegener's granulomatosis
c. Systemic lupus erythematosus
d. Thrombotic thrombocytopenic purpura

250. Postinfectious glomerulonephritis is characterized by which of the following?

a. Most cases in an epidemic are subclinical
b. Hematuria typically develops within a week of infection
c. More common with pharyngeal than cutaneous strep infection
d. Focal proliferative glomerulonephritis seen on renal biopsy
e. Children are often left with residual renal impairment

251. Which of the following is true of anti-GBM (glomerular basement membrane) syndrome?

a. The clinical presentation is largely the same in different age groups
b. The target antigen in the glomerulus is elastin
c. Complement levels are typically normal
d. Plasmapheresis enables dialysis-dependent patient to recover renal function
e. Transplantation is contraindicated because of disease recurrence

252. Prerenal azotemia is associated with

a. High fractional excretion of sodium
b. Granular casts in the urine
c. Use of angiotensin-converting enzyme (ACE) inhibitors in unilateral renal artery stenosis
d. Evolution to acute tubular necrosis if untreated

253. The pathologic findings of predominant small artery involvement with intimal proliferation and sometimes with thrombosis, also termed "thrombotic microangiopathy," is found in which renal disease?

a. Membranoproliferative glomerulonephritis
b. Hemolytic uremic syndrome
c. Microscopic polyarteritis
d. Analgesic nephropathy

254. Leukocytes and white cell casts in the urine are typically seen in

a. Radiocontrast nephropathy
b. Methicillin-induced renal insufficiency
c. Aminoglycoside nephrotoxicity
d. Rhabdomyolysis

255. Elevated anion gap and osmolar gap in a patient with renal failure suggests

a. ethylene glycol ingestion
b. isopropanol ingestion
c. mannitol infusion
d. radiocontrast administration

256. Which may cause acute renal failure in patients with nephrotic syndrome?

a. Dietary protein restriction
b. ACE inhibitors
c. Lipid-lowering agents
d. Loop diuretics

257. Hyponatremia with a low urine sodium is associated with

a. SIADH
b. congestive heart failure
c. recent thiazide use
d. hypothyroidism

258. Which disease presents with predominantly tubulointerstitial involvement?

a. Systemic lupus erythematosus
b. Sjögren's syndrome
c. Rheumatoid arthritis
d. Essential mixed cryoglobulinemia

259. Which disease presents with predominantly glomerular involvement?

a. Analgesic nephropathy
b. Uric acid nephropathy
c. Lead nephropathy
d. Light chain deposition disease

260. Which of the following patients would be better served by undergoing continuous ambulatory peritoneal dialysis rather than intermittent hemodialysis as treatment of chronic renal failure?

a. Patient with poor vision due to diabetic retinopathy
b. Patient with cardiomyopathy sensitive to fluid overload
c. Patient with severe COPD
d. Very obese patient

261. A patient on long-term lithium comes into your office complaining of polyuria; you would expect his serum sodium to be

a. Elevated because he has central diabetes insipidus
b. Elevated because he has nephrogenic diabetes insipidus
c. Nearly normal because he is drinking increased amounts of water
d. Low because he is suffering from psychogenic polydipsia

262. Concerning the association between potassium and bicarbonate abnormalities, which of the following is true?

a. The regulation of potassium excretion occurs largely in the loop of Henle, and this is why loop diuretics cause hypokalemia
b. Metabolic alkalosis is associated with volume depletion caused by diuretics
c. Hypokalemia generally results in the increased production of aldosterone
d. Volume depletion inhibits reabsorption of bicarbonate in the proximal tubule

263. Which of the following is characterized by normotension, hypo-kalemia, and metabolic alkalosis?

a. Sjögren's syndrome
b. Hyperaldosteronism
c. Liddle's syndrome
d. Barrter's syndrome

264. A 25-year-old man with flank pain is found to have three cysts in each kidney, normal hepatic and renal function, and family history is not clear. He is most likely to have

a. Autosomal dominant polycystic kidney disease
b. Autosomal recessive polycystic kidney disease
c. Acquired cystic disease
d. Medullary sponge kidney

265. Growth retardation, hypophosphatemia, and glycosuria may be associated with

a. Type 1 RTA
b. Type 2 RTA
c. Type 4 RTA
d. Diabetic nephropathy

266. Which is an accurate statement concerning diabetic nephropathy?

a. Most patients with type 2 diabetes will develop this problem
b. It is almost always associated with retinopathy in type 1 diabetes
c. ACE inhibition is only indicated for patients with hypertension
d. Routine dipstick urine should be performed to screen for early disease

267. Which of the following is a secondary cause for focal segmental sclerosis?

a. Hodgkin's disease
b. Colon cancer
c. HIV disease
d. Hepatitis C infection

268. A patient with Crohn's disease passes a kidney stone; the most likely composition is

a. Calcium phosphate
b. Uric acid
c. Struvite
d. Calcium oxalate

269. The metabolic disorder induced by diarrhea and by acetazolamide are best differentiated by

a. Serum anion gap
b. Blood gas analysis
c. Urine anion gap
d. Urine pH
e. Serum potassium

270. Which of the following would be a characteristic finding in obstructive nephropathy due to benign prostatic hypertrophy?

a. Hyperkalemia
b. Polyuria and nocturia
c. Hematuria
d. Suprapubic discomfort

271. Cirrhosis is a cause of

a. Hypervolemic hyponatremia
b. Isovolemic hyponatremia
c. Hypovolemic hyponatremia
d. Pseudohyponatremia

272. Which of the following statements characterizes minimal change disease?

a. It is associated with renal insufficiency despite treatment
b. It is associated with selective proteinuria
c. It is the most common cause of nephrotic syndrome in adults
d. It is diagnosed on light microscopy after kidney biopsy

273. Which of the following findings would favor essential hypertension over secondary hypertension?

a. Presence of hypokalemia and alkalosis
b. Presence of hyperinsulinemia and obesity
c. Presence of grade III fundoscopic findings
d. Presence of aortic aneurysm

274. A patient with long-standing COPD who develops vomiting would have which of the following blood gas and electrolyte patterns?

	Sodium	Chloride	Bicarbonate	pCO_2	pH
a.	139	105	25	38	7.44
b.	139	89	35	47	7.49
c.	140	95	25	40	7.42
d.	139	92	32	30	7.65

275. A patient with cardiomyopathy on chronic diuretics suffers acute respiratory arrest from aspiration has which of the following patterns?

	Sodium	Chloride	Bicarbonate	pCO_2	pH
a.	140	87	37	63	7.39
b.	140	104	26	60	7.26
c.	140	114	16	40	7.22
d.	140	96	33	75	7.26

276. A patient with diabetic ketoacidosis along with a bout of viral gastroenteritis resulting in diarrhea has which of the following patterns?

	Sodium	Chloride	Bicarbonate	pCO_2	pH
a.	140	109	12	26	7.29
b.	140	115	15	30	7.30
c.	140	103	15	25	7.34
d.	140	102	25	58	7.26

277. Hyperkalemia may be caused by

a. Trimethoprim
b. Albuterol
c. Licorice
d. Cisplatin

278. A middle-aged patient with an elevated serum creatinine, hypertension, and mild anemia comes to you for evaluation. Urine dipstick shows trace protein without red cells or cellular casts. A 24-h urine collection reveals 5 g of protein. The most likely etiology is

a. Focal segmental sclerosis
b. Hypertensive nephrosclerosis
c. Amyloidosis
d. Multiple myeloma

279. Which of the following is a common cause of isolated hematuria with isomorphic red cells in the urine?

a. Alport's syndrome (hereditary nephritis)
b. Thin basement membrane disease
c. Idiopathic hypercalciuria
d. IgA nephropathy

280. A 26-year-old woman with a history of mitral valve prolapse comes in with 1 week of fever that started 3 days after a dental procedure. Her urine contains red cells and her rheumatoid factor is elevated. Which of the following serologic abnormalities is expected to be present?

a. Anti-GBM antibody
b. Low serum complement levels
c. Antineutrophil cytoplasmic antibody
d. Elevated IgA levels

281. A 70-year-old man presents to you because he has not been feeling well for several months. He mainly complains of malaise and achiness. He takes ibuprofen occasionally for these symptoms. His urine shows protein and erythrocyte casts. A 24-h urine shows 1 g of protein per day. His creatinine clearance is 24 mL/min. About 4 months ago, his serum creatinine was normal. The most likely diagnosis is

a. Amyloidosis
b. Light chain deposition disease
c. Nonsteroidal induced interstitial nephritis
d. Vasculitis

Renal/Nephrology

Answers

237. The answer is a. *(Fauci, 14/e, p 1495.)* Pulmonary congestion due to fluid overload is a common finding in acute glomerulonephritis, which can resolve spontaneously as in postinfectious GN or lead to chronic renal failure as in lupus nephritis. Urinary findings consists of hematuria, red cell casts, and proteinuria. Leukocytes and eosinophils are seen in tubulointerstitial nephritis.

238. The answer is c. *(Fauci, 14/e, p 1496.)* The finding of broad casts reflects compensatory dilatation of surviving nephrons. Hyaline casts are a nonspecific finding. Proteinuria can be present in various stages of renal disease. Anemia and hypocalcemia can be present in acute renal failure and are usually multifactorial.

239. The answer is b. *(Fauci, 14/e, p 260.)* In nephrotic syndrome, the renin angiotensin system is activated, leading to salt and water retention and edema. Hyperlipidemia results from increased lipoprotein synthesis. Hypercoagulability results from loss of antithrombin III and reduced levels of proteins C and S. Although thyroid-binding globulin is lost, most patients are euthyroid when free T4 is measured.

240. The answer is d. *(Fauci, 14/e, p 1495.)* Hypocalcemia is due to decreased calcitrol synthesis and secondary hyperparathyroidism results. Bleeding time is prolonged due to uremic platelet inhibitors. Anemia is due to decreased erythropoietin synthesis. Hyperkalemia and hypermagnesemia is due to decreased excretion.

241. The answer is c. *(Fauci, 14/e, p 1508.)* In acute tubular necrosis, tubular damage prevents reabsorption of filtered sodium. In the other disorders listed, renal hypoperfusion causes avid sodium retention. Creatinine is not reabsorbed, hence leading to a low fractional excretion of sodium.

242. The answer is d. *(Fauci, 14/e, p 1500.)* Reabsorption of sodium and bicarbonate takes place largely in the proximal tubule. The loop of Henle is responsible for creating the hypertonicity of the medullary interstitium allowing for urinary concentration. Potassium regulation takes place in the distal tubule through the action of aldosterone and water regulation through ADH action in the collecting tubule.

243. The answer is d. *(Fauci, 14/e, p 1512.)* Metabolic acidosis is usually corrected if pH is less than 7.2. Hyperphosphatemia is managed initially with phosphate binders. Dopamine has not been shown to impact renal recovery. Hyponatremia is managed with water restriction. Hypervolemia is managed by decreasing salt and water intake and loop diuretics.

244. The answer is d. *(Fauci, 14/e, p 1516.)* Osteitis fibrosa is due to hyperparathyroidism and is associated with myopathy. Adynamic bone disease is associated with oversuppression of PTH. Osteomalacia is due to excessive aluminum accumulation. Amyloidosis in dialysis patients is due to β_2-microglobulin and not the amyloid proteins seen in usual amyloidosis. 1,25 dihydoxyvitamin D suppresses PTH production.

245. The answer is b. *(Fauci, 14/e, p 1518.)* Resistance to erythropoietin is most commonly due to iron deficiency despite oral iron intake. In a third of patients, the rise in hematocrit with erythropoietin therapy worsens with hypertension. Abnormal bleeding is treated with intensive dialysis, vasopressin, and estrogens among other measures but not with platelets. Although leukocyte function is impaired, sepsis is the second leading cause of death after cardiovascular disease.

246. The answer is d. *(Fauci, 14/e, p 1519.)* Erythropoietin is used to correct anemia of chronic renal failure. Most evidence suggests it does not hasten decline of renal function but is not protective. The other measures are recommended although protein restriction should be carefully monitored to avoid malnutrition.

247. The answer is c. *(Fauci, 14/e, p 1502.)* Adaptations to chronic renal insufficiency include increased fractional excretion of sodium due to hydraulic pressure, atrial natriuretic peptide, and vasodilatory prostaglandin; increased water excretion due to solute loss (osmotic diuresis); and metabolic acidosis due to retention of organic anions and decreased generation of ammonia. Potassium excretion is increased through augmented aldosterone production and extrarenal (i.e., colonic) losses.

248. The answer is a. *(Fauci, 14/e, p 1537.)* Anti-GBM disease is characterized by linear staining of the basement membrane. Immune complex disease, such as lupus or membranoproliferative glomerulonephritis is characterized by granular staining. ANCA-associated renal diseases were formerly called pauci-immune due to absence of staining by immunofluorescence.

249. The answer is b. *(Fauci, 14/e, p 1537.)* Goodpasture's syndrome consists of pulmonary hemorrhage and renal failure. The latter alone is called anti-GBM disease. ANCA is typically present in vasculitic disorders such as Wegener's, microscopic polyangiitis, and Churg-Strauss syndrome. SLE may have ANCA positivity if vasculitis is a prominent feature. TTP is primarily due to endothelial injury.

250. The answer is a. *(Fauci, 14/e, p 1539.)* Most cases of postinfectious GN are subclinical and found among contacts of the index case. Hematuria typically occurs 10 days or more after the infection, compared with IgA nephropathy in which the hematuria follows very closely thereafter. It is more common after cutaneous infection, unlike rheumatic fever, and the lesion is a diffuse proliferative glomerulonephritis. The prognosis in children is usually excellent.

251. The answer is c. *(Fauci, 14/e, p 1539.)* Complement levels are normal because it is not consumed in anti-GBM disease. Anti-GBM disease in the older age group is characterized by absence of pulmonary hemorrhage compared with the younger age group. The antigen is the NC1 domain of α-3 chain of type IV collagen. Although plasmapheresis is the treatment of choice, dialysis-dependent patients rarely recover renal function. Transplantation can be performed after seronegativity for a defined period with disease recurring only rarely.

252. The answer is d. *(Fauci, 14/e, p 1504.)* In prerenal azotemia, the renal dysfunction is initially reversible on restoration of renal perfusion but may evolve to tubular necrosis if the insult is not corrected. The urine sediment is bland and fractional excretion of sodium is low. Use of nonsteroidals or ACE inhibitors in predisposed patients, such as those with hypovolemia, heart failure, liver failure, or bilateral renal artery stenosis, may lead to prerenal azotemia.

253. The answer is b. *(Fauci, 14/e, p 1560.)* Thrombotic microangiopathy, which reflects predominantly endothelial injury in the small renal arterioles, is the hallmark of a group of diseases that includes hemolytic uremic syndrome, thrombotic thrombocytopenic purpura, scleroderma, sickle cell nephropathy, and malignant hypertension. This is the case because the primary process is endothelial damage.

254. The answer is b. *(Fauci, 14/e, p 1507.)* White cells and their casts are typically seen in pyelonephritis or acute interstitial nephritis such as seen with methicillin. Radiocontrast causes vasoconstriction and so the urinary sediment is bland. Aminoglycosides and rhabdomyolysis causes tubular necrosis and are associated with granular casts and renal tubular epithelial cell shedding in the urine.

255. The answer is a. *(Fauci, 14/e, p 1510.)* Only ethylene glycol and methanol ingestion present with an osmolar gap and metabolized to acids that cause an osmolar gap. Isopropanol and mannitol do not present with an anion gap.

256. The answer is d. *(Fauci, 14/e, p 1544.)* High-dose diuretics can precipitate acute renal failure in nephrotics because the intravascular volume cannot be defended by the hypoalbuminemia. The other three measures are generally considered helpful in nephrosis although dietary protein restriction needs monitoring to guard against malnutrition.

257. The answer is b. *(Fauci, 14/e, p 268.)* Hyponatremia associated with congestive heart failure is associated with low urine sodium due to decreased cardiac output and renal perfusion. Euvolemic hyponatremia, such as due to SIADH, hypothyroidism, or glucocorticoid deficiency, does not present with sodium retention. The main defect is free water excretion. Thiazide diuretics increase urine sodium loss.

258. The answer is b. *(Fauci, 14/e, p 1549.)* Sjögren's syndrome presents as a tubulointerstitial nephritis. Lupus may present with proliferative or membranous changes along with interstitial involvement. Rheumatoid arthritis usually presents with amyloidosis, whereas cryoglobulinemic nephropathy is a membranoproliferative lesion.

259. The answer is d. *(Fauci, 14/e, p 1555.)* Light chain deposition disease, found in paraproteinemias, presents with proteinuria and nephrotic syndrome due to glomerular deposition. The other diseases are examples of tubulointerstitial renal disease characterized by low albumin excretion in urine.

260. The answer is b. *(Fauci, 14/e, p 1523.)* Peritoneal dialysis is a daily treatment, and the gradual fluid removal is better tolerated by patients with poor cardiac reserve than hemodialysis. It requires adequate vision to be done independently. The abdominal distention may not be well tolerated by patients with COPD due to interference with lung expansion and the calories absorbed from dextrose-containing fluids may cause weight gain and obesity.

261. The answer is c. *(Fauci, 14/e, p 270.)* Lithium therapy results in nephrogenic diabetes insipidus. These patients maintain a high normal serum osmolarity unless water intake is restricted because the thirst center is intact and able to regulate serum osmolarity by water intake. They develop hypernatremia if they are hospitalized or develop CNS problems.

262. The answer is b. *(Fauci, 14/e, p 273.)* Potassium regulation takes place in the distal tubule and is regulated by aldosterone. Hypokalemia suppresses aldosterone production. Volume contraction increases proximal tubule bicarbonate reabsorption and leads to metabolic alkalosis.

263. The answer is d. *(Fauci, 14/e, p 273.)* Hyperaldosteronism (Conn's syndrome) is associated with hypertension, alkalosis, and hypokalemia due to increased aldosterone action. Liddle's syndrome, which is due to a mutation in the sodium channel, results in a similar picture. Sjögren's syndrome causes renal tubular acidosis and hypokalemia. Barrter's syndrome is due to a defect in a transporter in the loop of Henle and simulates a patient taking loop diuretics; because volume expansion does not occur, the patient is normotensive.

264. The answer is a. *(Fauci, 14/e, p 1563.)* Autosomal dominant PKD is diagnosed by ultrasound by the finding of three to five cysts in each kidney, especially in a young individual who is not expected to have acquired cystic disease (generally found in older individuals commonly with renal insufficiency). The recessive form leads to renal failure and hepatic fibrosis early in life. Medullary sponge kidney is autosomal dominant and diagnosed by IVP. It does not lead to renal failure.

265. The answer is b. *(Fauci, 14/e, p 1566.)* Type 1 RTA is a distal nephron disorder of acid excretion; nongap metabolic acidosis and hypokalemia ensues. Common causes include Sjögren's syndrome and hypergammaglobulinemia. Type 2 RTA is a proximal disorder of bicarbonate reclamation; it may be associated with Fanconi's syndrome (phosphate, amino acid, and glucose loss in the urine). Type 4 RTA presents with hyperkalemia and is caused by diabetes and tubulointerstitial nephropathy.

266. The answer is b. *(Fauci, 14/e, p 2076.)* About one-third of patients with diabetes will develop nephropathy. It is the most common cause of end-stage renal failure. It is nearly always associated with retinopathy in type 1 DM, but not in type 2 DM. Detection of microalbuminuria depends on 24-h urine collection or specialized urine dipsticks; the routine dipsticks are too insensitive. ACE inhibition may have a role in patients with microalbuminuria even before hypertension sets in.

267. The answer is c. *(Fauci, 14/e, p 1541.)* Glomerular lesions can be associated with systemic diseases. Common associations include minimal change with Hodgkin's disease and nonsteroidals; focal sclerosis with HIV infection, reflux nephropathy, and obesity; membranous nephropathy with hepatitis B, lupus, and solid tumors; and membranoproliferative lesions with hepatitis C and endocarditis.

268. The answer is d. *(Fauci, 14/e, p 1572.)* Inflammatory bowel disease causes fat malabsorption. The fat binds calcium, allowing oxalate absorption, leading to calcium oxalate stone formation. Calcium phosphate stones are formed by patients with renal tubular acidosis or hyperparathyroidism. Uric acid stones are associated with myeloproliferative syndromes or Lesch-Nyhan syndrome. Struvite stones are associated with infection.

269. The answer is c. *(Fauci, 14/e, p 1526.)* Both diarrhea and acetazolamide induce a nongap acidosis and hypokalemia. The urine pH is acidic (5.0) in diarrhea but is alkaline in acetazolamide administration only if the serum bicarbonate is above the threshold for complete reabsorption of bicarbonate (16 to 18 meq/L) The urine anion gap reliably differentiates renal from nonrenal causes of nongap acidosis.

270. The answer is b. *(Fauci, 14/e, p 1575.)* Chronic obstruction commonly results in polyuria and nocturia due to impaired urinary concentrating ability. Hyperkalemia is due to distal tubular damage. Hematuria should never be passed over as being due to BPH without further investigation. Because the process develops gradually, although the patient may complain of frequency and urgency, suprapubic discomfort is uncommon.

271. The answer is a. *(Fauci, 14/e, p 268.)* Congestive heart failure, cirrhosis, and nephrotic syndrome are causes of hypervolemic hyponatremia. Addison's disease and diuretic use lead to the hypovolemic form and SIADH is euvolemic. Pseudohyponatremia is associated with elevated lipids, glucose, or plasma proteins.

272. The answer is b. *(Fauci, 14/e, p 1541.)* Minimal change is the most common cause of nephrotic syndrome in children, but membranous nephropathy is more common in adults. The diagnosis is made by identifying foot process effacement on electron microscopy. By light microscopy, all findings are normal, hence the name "minimal change." Clinically, it is characterized by selective proteinuria principally due to loss of albumin and minimal amounts of higher molecular weight proteins, unlike in other diseases such as membranous glomerulopathy or focal sclerosis. It carries an excellent prognosis because remissions are typically obtained with steroid therapy.

273. The answer is b. *(Fauci, 14/e, p 1985.)* Secondary hypertension may be suggested by certain clues such as abrupt onset before the age of 25 years or after 50 years of age; abdominal bruits or signs of vascular disease such as an aneurysm; palpitations and tachycardia as in pheochromocytoma; hypokalemia and alkalosis as seen in hyperaldosteronism; and accelerated hypertension such as occurs in renal artery stenosis.

274. The answer is b. *(Fauci, 14/e, p 278.)* COPD produces a chronic respiratory acidosis that is compensated by a rise in serum bicarbonate. The vomiting introduces a metabolic alkalosis that further increases the serum bicarbonate. The relatively low bicarbonate in choices a. and c. suggests a preexisting metabolic acidosis, the former having a normal, and the latter an elevated anion gap. Choice d. suggests a combined metabolic and respiratory alkalosis.

275. The answer is d. *(Fauci, 14/e, p 278.)* This patient has an acute respiratory acidosis superimposed on a metabolic alkalosis caused by diuretics. Choice b. lacks the metabolic alkalosis, whereas choice c. lacks the respiratory acidosis; choice a. is more compatible with a chronic respiratory acidosis with the higher serum bicarbonate and nearly normal pH. The best choice is d.

276. The answer is a. *(Fauci, 14/e, p 278.)* This patient has a combined high anion gap and nongap metabolic acidosis, resulting in a fall in serum bicarbonate greater than the rise in the anion gap. The most compatible picture is a. Choice b. shows a nongap acidosis alone, and choice c. shows a gap acidosis alone. Choice d. shows a preexisting chronic respiratory acidosis.

277. The answer is a. *(Fauci, 14/e, p 275.)* Trimethoprim impairs potassium secretion in the distal nephron. Heparin, ACE inhibitors, and nonsteroidals are other examples of drugs that can cause hyperkalemia. The other three answers cause hypokalemia by cellular shifts (albuterol) or increased urinary loss (licorice, cisplatin).

278. The answer is d. *(Fauci, 14/e, p 1549.)* Urine dipstick cannot detect light chains and Bence Jones proteins found in paraproteinemias. So there is a discrepancy between dipstick values and the 24-h urine collection. The sulfosalicylic acid test (SSA) can precipitate all proteins and can be diagnostic as well. Focal sclerosis and amyloidosis would not have this discrepancy. Hypertensive nephrosclerosis presents with milder degrees of proteinuria.

279. The answer is c. *(Fauci, 14/e, p 1544.)* Glomerular diseases cause hematuria with dysmorphic red cells in the urine and sometimes red cell casts. Isomorphic red cells indicate nonglomerular bleeding including that from the urinary bladder. Hypercalciuria is a common cause of hematuria in young individuals even without renal stone formation.

280. The answer is b. *(Fauci, 14/e, p 1543.)* This clinical description is classic for membranoproliferative glomerulonephritis, which is associated with bacterial endocarditis. Choice a. describes anti-GBM antibody disease or Goodpasture's syndrome when the lung is involved. Choice c. describes pauci-immune glomerulonephritis, such as Wegener's. Choice d. describes IgA nephropathy. Low complement levels are typically found in membranoproliferative glomerulonephritis, but not in the other disorders listed.

281. The answer is d. *(Fauci, 14/e, p 1547.)* All of these diseases are common in older persons. Amyloidosis and light chain deposition disease are related to paraprotein deposition in the kidney and typically present with nephrotic syndrome. The subacute presentation and erythrocyte casts in the urine along with the rapid decline in renal function are most consistent with vasculitis. A positive antineutrophil cytoplasmic antibody (ANCA) would be supportive. Erythrocyte casts are not seen in the other diseases.

Gastroenterology

Questions

DIRECTIONS: Each item below contains a question or incomplete statement followed by suggested responses. Select the **one best** response to each question.

282. A 55-year-old man who is a longtime alcoholic comes to the emergency room after vomiting small amounts of bright red blood four times today. Your differential diagnosis is constructed around causes of bleeding from the

a. Colon
b. Liver and pancreas
c. Kidneys
d. Lungs
e. Upper gastrointestinal (GI) tract

283. A patient in your office tells you that he had an episode of vomiting bright red blood twice in 1 day about 1 week ago, followed the next day by three or four episodes of vomiting material that looked like coffee grounds. He could not afford to seek medical help then and he said that "it got better except for the pain." The past 3 days he noticed black "sticky" stools and he finally came to see you. What is your first concern?

a. Bleeding colon cancer
b. Bleeding from lung cancer
c. Crohn's disease
d. Cirrhosis
e. Bleeding peptic ulcer

284. A 60-year-old patient has epigastric pain and weight loss of a few pounds. The consulting gastroenterologist's evaluation includes upper GI endoscopy, and he discovers a gastric ulcer. Now, the gastroenterologist should

a. Biopsy the area of the ulcer
b. Cauterize the ulcer
c. Do nothing further
d. Consult a surgeon to do a partial gastrectomy
e. Repeat the upper GI endoscopy in 6 months

285. A 50-year-old woman executive has for the past 3 months experienced abdominal pain that often is relieved by antacids. Because of the persistent abdominal pain, she consults a gastroenterologist. He does an upper GI endoscopy and visualizes a duodenal ulcer. Now, the gastroenterologist should

a. Biopsy the ulcer
b. Arrange for a surgeon to operate on the ulcer
c. Suggest medical treatment of the ulcer
d. Cauterize the ulcer
e. Order an abdominal CT scan

286. A 70-year-old woman is evaluated with colonoscopy for anemia and intermittently hemoccult-positive stools. A diagnosis of multiple arteriovenous malformations (AVMs) is made by which diagnostic procedure?

a. Biopsy
b. Visual inspection
c. Arteriography
d. Venography
e. Lymphangiography

287. A 55-year-old alcoholic man has been losing weight for about 6 months and begins to complain of difficulty swallowing. An upper GI endoscopy reveals an esophageal ulcer. The gastroenterologist should

a. Biopsy the ulcerated area
b. Cauterize the ulcer
c. Do nothing further
d. Consult a surgeon to do an esophagectomy
e. Observe the patient and repeat the upper GI endoscopy in 6 months

288. A patient complaining of chest pain, regurgitation, and dysphagia for several months is thought to have achalasia. The gastroenterologist should

a. Order a chest CT scan to rule out tracheoesophageal fistula
b. Do an endoscopy to biopsy the lower esophageal sphincter
c. Do an endoscopy to dilate the esophagus
d. Do an endoscopy to inject botulinum toxin into the lower esophageal sphincter
e. Order an abdominal CT scan to make the diagnosis of achalasia

289. Hepatitis C virus is most commonly transmitted by

a. Parenteral routes including intravenous drug abuse and promiscuous sex
b. Fecal-oral route
c. Ingestion of contaminated food or water
d. Living in the same household as an infected person
e. Inhalation of infected airborne particles

290. The percentage of patients with acute hepatitis C who go on to have chronic disease is

a. 5 to 10
b. 15 to 20
c. 25 to 30
d. 40 to 50
e. 60 to 70

291. The extent of liver damage done by chronic hepatitis B or C infection can best be gauged by evaluating

a. Symptoms
b. Elevation of serum transaminases
c. Duration of infection
d. Liver biopsy
e. Presence or absence of ascites

292. A 45-year-old obese woman with cholelithiasis presents to the emergency room complaining of nausea and vomiting for 2 days, along with severe continuous midabdominal pain. She has a low-grade fever and the ER physician finds that she has a slightly elevated WBC count (12,000) and an elevated serum amylase. The most likely diagnosis is

a. Ruptured abdominal aortic aneurysm
b. Hepatitis
c. Peptic ulcer disease
d. Early phase of acute appendicitis
e. Acute pancreatitis

293. Chronic pancreatitis may be reliably diagnosed in a patient presenting with

a. Calcification in the pancreas detected on a flat plate x-ray of the abdomen
b. Abdominal pain
c. Diarrhea
d. Nausea and vomiting
e. Jaundice

294. Acute pancreatitis is caused by a variety of disorders. Which of the following pairs of disorders account for 80 to 90% of cases?

a. Diabetes and viral illness
b. Trauma and hyperlipidemia
c. Trauma and gallstones
d. Hyperlipidemia and alcohol
e. Alcohol and gallstones

295. A 70-year-old man with progressive painless jaundice is referred to your office. You order liver function tests that show an abnormal pattern consistent with obstruction. Which procedure will you now suggest?

a. Laparoscopic cholecystectomy
b. Endoscopic retrograde cholangiopancreatography (ERCP)
c. Modified barium swallow
d. Laparoscopic abdominal exploration
e. Upper GI endoscopy

296. In which of the following disorders will esophageal manometry reveal a high-pressure nonrelaxing LES and poor motility in the rest of the esophagus?

a. Hypertensive LES
b. Esophageal spasm
c. Obstructive lower esophageal lesion
d. Nonspecific motility disorders
e. Achalasia

297. A 70-year-old man complains of a sensation of food sticking in his lower chest area. This happens when he eats either liquids or solids. He also has a slight weight loss. The most likely diagnosis is

a. Achalasia
b. Esophageal spasm
c. Hypertensive LES
d. Hiatal hernia with GERD
e. Barrett's esophagus

298. A 45-year-old woman has chest pain for which a cardiac cause has been ruled out. Her esophageal motility study shows pressure waves of a very high amplitude lasting 2 to 3 s. The most likely diagnosis is

a. Esophageal web
b. Esophageal spasm
c. Achalasia
d. GERD (gastroesophageal reflux disease)
e. T-E (tracheoesophageal) fistula

299. A 40-year-old man with occasional dysphagia and who otherwise feels well undergoes esophageal motility studies that show an LES amplitude of approximately 60 mmHg. The esophagus relaxes completely when he swallows. The most likely diagnosis is

a. GERD (gastroesophageal reflux disease)
b. Achalasia
c. Hypertensive LES
d. Barrett's esophagus
e. Esophageal spasm

300. The presence of gastroesophageal reflux is best diagnosed by

a. Computed tomographic (CT) scan of the chest
b. Physical examination
c. Laboratory evaluation
d. Barium swallow
e. Medical history

301. The most common location for a gastric ulcer is

a. Fundus
b. Greater curvature
c. Cardia
d. Body
e. Antrum

302. *Helicobacter pylori* is associated with

a. Nearly all duodenal ulcers and most gastric ulcers
b. Few peptic ulcers
c. Most esophageal ulcers, but not many gastric ulcers
d. Nearly all gastric ulcers, but very few duodenal ulcers
e. Most cases of erosive gastritis

303. When nonsteroidal anti-inflammatory drugs cause ulcers, they are usually

a. Esophageal
b. Jejunal
c. Duodenal
d. Gastric
e. Anal

304. A 40-year-old man comes to your office complaining of epigastric pain that is unrelieved by several weeks of antacid therapy. Endoscopy reveals a duodenal ulcer. You recommend a course of treatment. What is the most likely outcome?

a. The ulcer may heal but scarring will cause outlet obstruction
b. Eventually the patient will require surgery for control of his symptoms
c. The ulcer may heal completely after 8 weeks of H2-blocker therapy
d. The symptoms will improve with H2-blocker therapy, but the ulcer won't heal
e. The ulcer may heal completely after 6 months of H2-blocker therapy

305. Which one of these ulcers has the lowest incidence of malignancy?

a. Duodenal
b. Esophageal
c. Gastric
d. Colon
e. Gastroesophageal junction

306. Osmolality of bowel contents under normal circumstances is

a. Isotonic in the jejunum, ileum, and colon and variable in the duodenum
b. Variable throughout the small and large intestines
c. Isotonic in the colon and hypertonic in the small intestine
d. Hypertonic throughout the small and large intestines
e. Variable in the jejunum, ileum, and colon and isotonic in the duodenum

307. The digestive enzymes amylase and lipase begin to be secreted and begin to act on ingested food

a. In the duodenum, after they are secreted by the pancreas
b. In the ileum, after they are secreted by the small intestine
c. In the duodenum, after they are secreted from the liver
d. In the mouth, after secretion from the salivary and lingual glands
e. In the stomach, after they are secreted from the pancreas

308. A 72-year-old woman complains of fatigue, dyspepsia, and shortness of breath. Her daughter tells you that her mother also has some slight memory loss and occasionally complains of numbness in her legs. The laboratory tests you ordered show a hemoglobin of 10.2 g/dL and an MCV of 110. The most likely cause is

a. Autoantibodies to thyroglobulin
b. Autoantibodies to histones
c. Autoantibodies to gastric parietal cells
d. Autoantibodies to dsDNA (double-stranded DNA)
e. Autoantibodies to ribosomal P protein

309. A 45-year-old man complains of frequent "heartburn" and a mild chronic cough. On examination, he has gastroesophageal reflux disease (GERD). In addition to prescribing medications, which one of the following dietary recommendations would you make?

a. Avoid high-protein meals because they would increase lower esophageal sphincter (LES) pressure
b. Avoid fats, chocolates, and alcohol because they would decrease LES pressure
c. Eat high-carbohydrate food to increase overall GI motility
d. Eat high-protein meals to decrease LES pressure
e. Avoid concentrated carbohydrates to decrease dopamine secretion

310. A 32-year-old man is admitted with a bleeding ulcer. This is his fifth episode of bleeding from gastric ulcers and he also has moderate diarrhea. Each time, his ulcers have been difficult to resolve. Which neoplastic lesion is most likely to be found in this man?

a. Small cell carcinoma of the lung
b. Gastric adenocarcinoma
c. Small intestinal carcinoid
d. Prostate adenocarcinoma
e. Gastrinoma

311. Which clinical or laboratory finding is most consistently seen in malabsorption syndromes?

a. Hypercalcemia
b. Iron overload
c. Elevated zinc levels in serum
d. Normal small bowel biopsy
e. Steatorrhea

312. In which disorder is malabsorption due to diminished or absent digestive enzymes?

a. Chronic pancreatitis
b. Crohn's disease
c. Gastric surgery
d. Small bowel ischemia
e. Sigmoid resection

313. A 35-year-old woman has had episodes of abdominal pain and bloody diarrhea for 4 to 5 years. Recently, the episodes became increasingly common, and she noted a weight loss of about 10 pounds. She tells you that two of her uncles have had similar symptoms "for years" and recently one of them had colon cancer. On examination, there are no abdominal masses and no fistulas. The most likely findings on colonoscopy with biopsy are

a. Normal mucosa
b. Patchy inflammatory lesions that extend throughout the bowel wall
c. Granulomas and fibrosis
d. Continuous inflammatory changes mostly confined to the mucosa
e. Patchy inflammation of the mucosa with inflamed mesenteric fat and fibrosis

314. A 20-year-old man has complaints of diarrhea and abdominal pain. He often sees some blood in his stool, but not with every episode of diarrhea. He also complains of easy fatigue and weight loss and for 2 days he has had nausea and vomiting. Two years ago he was treated for a rectal fissure. On examination, he has a modestly tender mass in the right lower quadrant. The most likely diagnosis is

a. Ulcerative colitis
b. Appendicitis
c. Diverticulitis
d. Irritable bowel syndrome
e. Crohn's disease

315. You suspect a patient may have gallstones as a cause of her chronic nausea and mild RUQ pain. The best imaging study would be

a. Upper abdominal ultrasound
b. Abdominal CT scan
c. Abdominal MRI
d. Barium swallow
e. KUB (flat-plate x-ray of the abdomen)

316. A patient with jaundice complains of RUQ pain. Liver function tests show a bilirubin of 3.0 mg/dL, alkaline phosphatase about four times normal and both AST and ALT increased about 50% above normal. The best imaging test to order first in evaluating this patient would be

a. Ultrasound
b. Abdominal CT scan
c. Abdominal MRI
d. Barium swallow
e. KUB (flat-plate x-ray of the abdomen)

317. A patient with colon cancer diagnosed about 2 years ago presents with slight jaundice, nausea, and weight loss. An abdominal CT scan is read as "lesions in the liver; unable to distinguish vascular from possible metastatic areas." What is the best imaging study for this patient?

a. Upper abdominal ultrasound
b. Repeat CT scan with spiral technique
c. Abdominal MRI
d. Laparoscopy
e. Open abdominal exploration

318. A 65-year-old man complains of "trouble swallowing." He is unsure whether his "trouble swallowing" occurs with both liquids and solids because it is intermittent. Sometimes he "chokes" and gets food "in his windpipe." The best imaging study is

a. Ultrasound of the neck
b. CT scan of the chest
c. MRI of the mediastinum
d. Barium swallow
e. KUB (flat-plate x-ray of the abdomen)

319. Symptoms due to *Clostridium difficile* infection can be accurately diagnosed by

a. Presence of diarrhea
b. Stool positive for WBCs
c. History of recent antibiotic usage
d. Pseudomembranes noted on a sigmoidoscopy
e. KUB (flat-plate x-ray of the abdomen)

320. Which term characterizes the frequency of chronic disease following hepatitis A infection?

a. Rare
b. Infrequent
c. Common
d. Typical
e. Nonexistent

321. Which of the following laboratory patterns is most consistent with the diagnosis of hemochromatosis?

a. Increased iron, increased TIBC (total iron-binding capacity), and increased ferritin
b. Low iron, low TIBC, and low ferritin
c. Low iron, low TIBC, and increased ferritin
d. Low iron, increased TIBC, and decreased ferritin
e. Increased iron, normal TIBC, and low ferritin

322. Which of the following is seen most commonly in association with primary biliary cirrhosis (PBC)?

a. Positive antinuclear antibody (ANA)
b. Increased ceruloplasmin
c. Increased ferritin
d. Positive hepatitis B surface antigen
e. Positive antimitochondrial antibody (AMA)

323. Previously, you treated a 44-year-old man, a former intravenous drug abuser, for acute hepatitis C infection. Several months later, it is clear that the patient has chronic hepatitis and may need therapy with interferon. Which long-term complications of hepatitis C infection must you discuss so that the patient can make an informed decision about treatment?

a. Hepatoma and cirrhosis
b. Hepatic adenoma
c. Sclerosing cholangitis
d. Hemochromatosis
e. Lymphoma or leukemia

324. Fatigue, anorexia, orange/brown-colored urine, and an ALT level greater than 10 times normal are clinical features of

a. Hepatitis A
b. Any viral hepatitis
c. Hepatoma
d. Hepatitis B and hepatitis C
e. Hepatitis B, but not hepatitis C

325. Protective vaccines are available for which of the following hepatitis viruses?

a. A and B
b. A and D
c. A and C
d. B and C
e. C and D

326. A man known to be an alcoholic for at least 15 years presents with fever, elevated serum bilirubin, elevated WBC count, and an AST/ALT ratio greater than 2. A liver biopsy shows Mallory bodies, WBCs, and degenerating cells. You should tell this patient that the biopsy findings are

a. Consistent with cirrhosis
b. Essentially normal
c. Consistent with alcoholic hepatitis that may revert to normal if he stops drinking alcohol
d. Consistent with alcoholic hepatitis that will progress to cirrhosis
e. Not interpretable because of the presence of degenerating cells and it will need to be repeated

Gastroenterology

Answers

282. The answer is e. *(Fauci, 14/e, p 246.)* Hematemesis or vomiting of blood represents an upper gastrointestinal (GI) source of blood loss. Bleeding from the colon will be manifested by either by no change in the color of the stools or by black, tarry-like stools (melena). Bleeding from the lungs results in blood in the sputum (hemoptysis) and from the kidneys as blood in the urine (hematuria), mainly microscopic hematuria.

283. The answer is e. *(Fauci, 14/e, p 1607.)* Vomiting of blood or hematemesis can be either fresh, bright red blood or dark blood (similar to coffee grounds in appearance), which results from the action of gastric chemicals on the blood. Blood that appears as coffee grounds signals bleeding from the stomach or duodenum. Tarry or black stools occur with bleeding from the colon. It can occur also with substantial amounts of bleeding from the upper gastrointestinal tract, such as bleeding from a peptic ulcer.

284. The answer is a. *(Fauci, 14/e, pp 518, 1607.)* Gastric ulcers should be biopsied to rule out malignancy. The other approaches are not appropriate.

285. The answer is c. *(Fauci, 14/e, pp 568, 1607.)* The incidence of malignancy in duodenal ulcer is low, so a biopsy of the ulcer is not indicated. Surgery or other procedures are not necessary in uncomplicated ulcers.

286. The answer is b. *(Fauci, 14/e, pp 568, 1607.)* AVMs are recognized visually and no biopsies are necessary. This is so particularly because of the increased incidence of bleeding.

287. The answer is a. *(Fauci, 14/e, pp 568, 1607.)* Like gastric ulcers, esophageal ulcers should always be biopsied because ulcerating lesions of the esophagus on contrast radiographs can be cancer. Esophageal cancers are mainly squamous cell carcinomas. Although uncommon, esophageal cancer is particularly aggressive and less than 5% of persons survive 5 years.

288. The answer is d. *(Fauci, 14/e, pp 1590.)* In achalasia, the esophagus is dilated, sometimes significantly so to the point of mimicking the sigmoid. Endoscopy with injection of botulinin toxin into the LES may be useful, and it would provide a direct view of the dilation. Biopsy is not necessary unless the mucosal surface is irregular.

289. The answer is a. *(Fauci, 14/e, pp 1686.)* Hepatitis C requires parenteral exposure for transmission. It is most commonly spread through intravenous drug abuse. It also spread by sexual contact; however, this occurs very infrequently.

290. The answer is e. *(Fauci, 14/e, pp 1690.)* Up to 75% of patients infected with hepatitis C subsequently may become carriers and develop chronic disease. Interferon and ribavirin in combination cure about 40% of persons with HCV serotype 1a and about 60% of persons with HCV serotype 3a.

291. The answer is d. *(Fauci, 14/e, pp 1700.)* Obtaining a piece of liver tissue is the only means to judge the histologic damage caused by chronic viral infection. A poor correlation exists between symptoms and transaminase elevation, as well as the duration of infection and liver damage.

292. The answer is e. *(Fauci, 14/e, pp 1581.)* The characteristics of acute pancreatitis include nausea and vomiting, abdominal pain, low-grade fever, and an elevated serum amylase. The pain is located primarily in the epigastrium and radiates into the back and usually is continuous and boring in quality. Fever may or may not be present. Serum amylase and lipase are usually elevated in the acute stages.

293. The answer is a. *(Fauci, 14/e, pp 1741.)* Jaundice, abdominal pain, diarrhea, and nausea and vomiting all occur in patients suffering from chronic pancreatitis, but these findings are nonspecific. The finding of calcification on the KUB (kidneys, ureters, and bladder) or flat-plate x-ray is diagnostic of chronic pancreatitis.

294. The answer is e. *(Fauci, 14/e, pp 1741.)* Gallstones and alcohol-induced disease account for 80 to 90% of the cases of acute pancreatitis. Less common causes include trauma, viral illnesses, hypercalcemia, and medications. Diabetes is not a cause of acute pancreatitis.

295. The answer is b. *(Fauci, 14/e, pp 1584.)* Therapeutic ERCP is used most commonly for complicated gallstone disease, as well as for an evaluation of obstructive jaundice. It can nonsurgically relieve obstructive jaundice. When needed, during ERCP sphincterotomy can be performed or stents usually can be placed very safely, with an approximately 5% complication rate. Most complications are not serious.

296. The answer is e. *(Fauci, 14/e, pp 1741.)* Achalasia shows a high-pressure nonrelaxing LES with absent motility in the body of the esophagus. Hypertensive LES has a high-pressure reading at the LES. Esophageal spasm shows high-amplitude prolonged pressure waves. Nonspecific disorders include repetitive swallows and dropped waves that do move through the whole esophagus. Obstructive causes of dysphagia are best diagnosed on barium swallow or endoscopy.

297. The answer is a. *(Fauci, 14/e, pp 1741.)* Patients with achalasia present with a history of dysphagia or sensation of food sticking, which includes both liquids and solids. They have a long history of these symptoms and might come for treatment at an older age.

298. The answer is b. *(Fauci, 14/e, pp 1741.)* Patients with esophageal spasm usually have more severe pain than patients with hypertensive (hypercontracting) LES (and the other disorders). The symptoms of esophageal spasm often are confused with the pain of cardiac origin. Patients with esophageal spasm and hypertensive (hypercontracting) LES usually present at an earlier age than patients with achalasia.

299. The answer is c. *(Fauci, 14/e, pp 1590–1591.)* Patients with hypertensive (hypercontracting) LES experience less dysphagia than patients with esophageal spasm, and they do not complain of food sticking as do patients with achalasia. The pain associated with hypertensive LES does not have the characteristic of cardiac origin.

300. The answer is e. *(Fauci, 14/e, pp 1593.)* The diagnosis of gastroesophageal reflux is best diagnosed by a medical history because of its typical presentation of retrosternal burning, usually postprandially and sometimes nocturnally. It may be exacerbated by certain foods. In simple reflux disease, the results of a physical examination and laboratory tests are unremarkable. CT findings of the chest are normal in reflux disease. Gastroesophageal reflux can be elicited on barium swallow, but often it is only an incidental and unrelated finding in patients who have no symptoms of heartburn.

301. The answer is e. (*Fauci, 14/e, pp 1593.*) Eighty-five to 90% of gastric ulcers are found in the prepyloric and antral areas. An ulcer in a different location is unusual, but it is not indicative of a higher incidence of malignancy.

302. The answer is a. (*Fauci, 14/e, pp 1605.*) *Helicobacter pylori* is associated as a cause of approximately 95% of duodenal ulcers and 75% of gastric ulcers. It is also universally associated with antral gastritis. About one-half of the adult population in the U.S. harbors *Helicobacter pylori*. However, in adults it rarely causes symptoms.

303. The answer is d. (*Fauci, 14/e, pp 1605.*) Nonsteroidal anti-inflammatory drugs primarily cause gastric ulcers. They also can cause duodenal disease. Because of the concern for malignancy in gastric ulcers, biopsies are performed of gastric ulcers to search for malignant changes.

304. The answer is c. (*Fauci, 14/e, pp 1605.*) After only 8 weeks of H2-blocker therapy, the ulcer may heal. Six months of H2-blocker will not prove more beneficial than 6 weeks of such therapy and it is not indicated. Symptoms lessen because the ulcer heals. Surgery is rarely indicated for the control of symptoms, considering the high efficacy of the medications currently available. Duodenal ulcers are at exceedingly low risk for any malignancy; therefore, biopsies of them are not routinely performed.

305. The answer is a. (*Fauci, 14/e, pp 1605.*) Duodenal ulcers are at exceedingly low risk for any malignancy, unlike the other ulcers. Gastric ulcers especially show malignancy.

306. The answer is a. (*McPhee, 2/e, p 293.*) The duodenum has the highest fluid flow rate and the most variable osmolality of any area in the intestinal tract. Its flow rate exceeds any area in the small and large intestine.

307. The answer is d. (*McPhee, 2/e, p 293.*) Digestion begins in the mouth with the action of chewing. Amylase from the salivary glands and lipase from the lingual glands start to act in the mouth.

308. The answer is c. *(McPhee, 2/e, pp 290; Fauci, 14/e, pp 655, 656, 1875, 2018.)* The syndrome described is most consistent with pernicious anemia, a macrocytic anemia, in which 90% of persons with this disease have antibodies to gastric parietal cells and about 60% of persons possess anti-intrinsic factor antibody. The antiparietal cell antibody destroys parietal cells and leads to malabsorption of cobalamin and a macrocytic anemia. Antibodies to histones, dsDNA, and ribosomal P protein occur in systemic lupus erythematosus (SLE). Autoantibodies to thyroglobulin are characteristic of Hashimoto's disease.

309. The answer is b. *(McPhee, 2/e, pp 296.)* The goal for improving the symptoms of GERD is to increase or maintain the LES pressure. High-protein meals generally increase LES pressure and should be encouraged. Fats, chocolate, and alcohol decrease LES pressure and these foods should be avoided. Carbohydrate content does not affect motility.

310. The answer is e. *(McPhee, 2/e, p 240; Fauci, 14/e, p 1614.)* The clinical findings in this patient are consistent with a diagnosis of Zollinger-Ellison syndrome (multiple peptic ulcers due to a gastrin-secreting tumor). Diarrhea accompanies the symptoms of peptic ulcer frequently. The patient is a young adult and lacks other symptoms of a gastric adenocarcinoma. Carcinoid causes diarrhea, but not often does it cause the ulcerative symptoms this patient exhibits. Also, this patient's symptoms are inconsistent with lung or prostate carcinoma.

311. The answer is e. *(Fauci, 14/e, pp 1619–1620.)* The presence of steatorrhea is diagnostic for malabsorption particularly when more than 6 g of fat is excreted per day. Villous atrophy on small bowel biopsy specimens is consistent also with changes leading to malabsorption. Calcium and iron are not absorbed well in the upper small intestine, and their levels are low. Similarly, the zinc level should be low.

312. The answer is a. *(Fauci, 14/e, p 1621.)* The causes of malabsorption include the absence of digestive enzymes (as occurs in chronic pancreatitis) or injured or absent small bowel mucosa (as occurs in Crohn's disease, various gastric surgeries, and ischemia resulting in bowel resection.) Sigmoid resection or removal of all or part of the colon should not impair absorption of nutrients.

313. The answer is d. *(Fauci, 14/e, p 1637–1639.)* Ulcerative colitis usually shows continuous inflammatory changes mostly confined to the mucosa of the colon without skip lesions. Granulomas are not seen in biopsy specimens. Clinically, diarrhea, frequently bloody, characterizes ulcerative colitis. After 10 years of total colonic involvement, an increased risk exists of colon malignancy.

314. The answer is e. *(McPhee, 2/e, p 315; Fauci, 14/e, p 1637–1639.)* Crohn's disease can present confined to the small bowel or colon or more commonly with a combination of ileocolonic involvement. It frequently has skip lesions throughout the small bowel and colon, with abnormal mucosa separated by normal mucosa. It can present with nausea and vomiting, secondary to obstruction due to fibrosing disease, stricture, or abscess.

315. The answer is a. *(Fauci, 14/e, pp 253–255, 1664.)* An upper abdominal ultrasound is the ideal test to examine the gallbladder for stones. CT scan is very helpful in evaluating obstructive jaundice, particularly when a pancreatic source is suspected. For subtle lesions for which the differential diagnosis includes metastatic disease, vascular problems, or parenchymal disease, MRI is very helpful if the CAT scan is not diagnostic. Barium swallow is the initial study favored in the evaluation of patients with dysphagia. A KUB can show radiopaque stones only.

316. The answer is b. *(Fauci, 14/e, pp 253–255, 1664.)* CT scan is very helpful in evaluating obstructive jaundice, particularly when a pancreatic source is suspected. For subtle lesions for which the differential diagnosis includes metastatic disease, vascular problems, or parenchymal disease, MRI is very helpful if the CAT scan is not diagnostic. An upper abdominal ultrasound is the ideal test to examine the gallbladder for stones, and a barium swallow is the initial study favored in the evaluation of patients with dysphagia. A KUB might show an enlarged liver, but contribute to the evaluation of jaundice, especially when the pancreas is involved.

317. The answer is c. *(Fauci, 14/e, pp 253–255, 1664.)* For subtle lesions for which the differential diagnosis includes metastatic disease, vascular problems, or parenchymal disease, MRI is very helpful if the CAT scan is not diagnostic. An upper abdominal ultrasound is the ideal test to examine the gallbladder for stones. CT scan is very helpful in evaluating obstructive jaundice, particularly when a pancreatic source is suspected.

318. The answer is d. *(Fauci, 14/e, pp 253–255, 1664.)* Barium swallow is the initial study favored in the evaluation of patients with dysphagia. An ultrasound of the neck will not provide information on dysphagia with difficulty swallowing liquids and solids because the lesion causing this symptom is in the esophagus.

319. The answer is d. *(Fauci, 14/e, p 909.)* The diagnosis of *Clostridium difficile* infection can be made accurately by the presence of pseudomembranes on sigmoidoscopy and also by identifying *C. difficile* toxins in the stools. The presence of diarrhea and WBCs in the stool are not specific and not diagnostic of *C. difficile,* which usually are seen with prior antibiotic usage, but these findings are not totally reliable.

320. The answer is e. *(Fauci, 14/e, p 1684.)* Patients with acute hepatitis A do not progress to chronic disease, unlike those patients infected with hepatitis B or hepatitis C viruses. In acute hepatitis A, the case fatality rate is less than 1%, and there is no chronic disease secondary to it.

321. The answer is a. *(Fauci, 14/e, p 1251.)* The findings of an increased serum iron, slightly increased TIBC, and increased ferritin level is consistent with the diagnosis of hemochromatosis. The increased ferritin level is usually greater than 500. Low iron, low TIBC, and low ferritin are not characteristic of hemochromatosis.

322. The answer is e. *(Fauci, 14/e, p 1621.)* Positive AMA is seen in approximately 95% of primary biliary cirrhosis (PBC) patients. ANA is seen in a few patients. Decreased ceruloplasmin and increased ferritin levels are usually seen in Wilson's disease and hemochromatosis, respectively. There is no association between Hepatitis B surface antigen and PBC.

323. The answer is a. *(Fauci, 14/e, p 1699.)* The most serious consequences of chronic hepatitis B and C infections are hepatoma and cirrhosis. Complications of cirrhosis may occur, resulting in liver failure. Chronic hepatitis is not a risk factor for adenoma, cholangitis, lymphoma, or hemochromatosis.

324. The answer is b. *(Fauci, 14/e, p 1677.)* Acute viral hepatitis, no matter what the etiology, usually presents in a similar manner with fatigue and anorexia, malaise, and dark-colored urine, if jaundice is present. The transaminases, AST and ALT, are usually elevated 10 times above normal levels.

325. The answer is a. *(Fauci, 14/e, p 1705.)* Currently, protective vaccines are available for hepatitis A (2 doses 6 months apart) and hepatitis B (3 doses; second dose follows the first by 1 month and third dose follows the second dose by 5 months). No vaccines exist for other hepatitis viruses.

326. The answer is c. *(Fauci, 14/e, p 1705.)* Acute alcoholic hepatitis is characterized by the presence of Mallory bodies and WBCs in the liver biopsy specimen. Frequently, it shows fat and degenerating cells in the liver. Usually, with abstinence from alcohol, this will revert to a normal histologic pattern. However, on occasion, liver disease can progress despite abstinence.

Liver Disease

Questions

DIRECTIONS: Each item below contains a question or incomplete statement followed by suggested responses. Select the **one best** response to each question.

327. Serum alkaline phosphatase may be elevated in the diseases of which organ?

a. Liver
b. Salivary glands
c. Spleen
d. Heart
e. Bladder

328. In parenchymal liver disease, which one of the following tests of liver function likely will be decreased from normal?

a. AST (aspartate aminotransferase) and ALT (alanine aminotransferase)
b. Alkaline phosphatase
c. Albumin
d. Prothrombin time
e. γ-Glutamyl transpeptidase (GGT)

329. In obstructive liver disease, which one of the following tests of liver function likely remains normal?

a. AST and ALT
b. Alkaline phosphatase
c. Albumin
d. 5′-Nucleotidase
e. γ-Glutamyl transpeptidase (GGT)

330. Which one of the following enzymes is found primarily in the liver?

a. AST
b. ALT
c. Alkaline phosphatase
d. 5′-Nucleotidase
e. γ-Glutamyl transpeptidase (GGT)

331. A 43-year-old woman comes to your office complaining of pruritus, mainly of the soles and palms, and fatigue. She has minimal jaundice and steatorrhea. Laboratory tests show a slightly elevated bilirubin, an elevated alkaline phosphatase, and a positive IgG antimitochondrial antibody test. The likely diagnosis is

a. Extrahepatic biliary tract obstruction
b. Alcoholic hepatitis
c. Viral hepatitis
d. Primary biliary cirrhosis
e. Carcinoma of the liver

332. Transmission of hepatitis A is almost exclusively by

a. Blood transfusion
b. Intravenous drug abuse
c. Fecal-oral route
d. Sexual

333. Which one of the hepatitis viruses is a DNA virus?

a. HAV
b. HBV
c. HCV
d. HEV
e. HGV

334. In hepatitis B virus infection, which one of the following antibodies is the protective antibody?

a. Anti-HBe
b. Anti-HBc
c. Anti-HBs
d. Anti-polymerase
e. Anti-HBV DNA

335. A 51-year-old man health care worker whom you examine for the first time feels well. You do a complete physical examination, which is normal except for slight overweight and borderline hypertension. It is interesting that his laboratory studies show the following hepatitis B virus profile: positive HBsAg, negative anti-HBs, low levels of IgG anti-HBc, positive anti-HBeAg, and negative anti-HBe. The likely diagnosis is

a. Acute HBV infection, high infectivity
b. Late-acute HBV, low infectivity
c. Recovered from HBV infection
d. Chronic HBV infection, high infectivity
e. Immunization with HBsAg vaccine

336. A 55-year-old woman manager of a regional long-distance telephone office whom you examine for the first time feels well. You do a complete physical examination, which is normal except for a few very small palpable and moveable, nontender nodes in both cervical chains and occasional wheezes in the lungs. However, her laboratory studies show the following hepatitis B virus profile: negative HBsAg, positive anti-HBs, low levels of IgG anti-HBc, negative anti-HBeAg, and positive anti-HBe. The likely diagnosis is

a. Acute HBV infection, high infectivity
b. Late-acute HBV, low infectivity
c. Recovered from HBV infection
d. Chronic HBV infection, high infectivity
e. Immunization with HBsAg vaccine

337. The most common cause of fulminant hepatitis is hepatitis

a. A
b. B
c. C
d. E
e. G

338. Mallory bodies found on biopsy of the liver are highly suggestive of which disease?

a. Alcoholic fatty liver
b. Alcoholic hepatitis
c. Alcoholic cirrhosis
d. Viral hepatitis
e. Primary biliary cirrhosis

339. A 26-year-old man comes to your office for an examination because of tremors, spasticity, and drooling. He has headaches and fatigue. On physical examination, he is very slightly icteric, the liver is not palpable, and no spider angiomata are present, but he has resting and intention tremors and spasticity. Laboratory tests show elevated AST and ALT and a ceruloplasmin level of 70 mg/L. The diagnosis is

a. Hemochromatosis
b. Gaucher's disease
c. Biliary cirrhosis
d. Wilson's disease
e. Type III glycogen storage disease

340. Which of these liver diseases results from a copper disorder?

a. Hemochromatosis
b. Gaucher's disease
c. Biliary cirrhosis
d. Wilson's disease
e. Type III glycogen storage disease

341. Which of these liver diseases results from an iron disorder?

a. Hemochromatosis
b. Gaucher's disease
c. Biliary cirrhosis
d. Wilson's disease
e. Type III glycogen storage disease

342. Which feature characterizes acetaminophen-induced liver damage?

a. Fatal fulminant disease usually is associated with ingestion of 25 g or more of acetaminophen
b. Blood levels of acetaminophen fail to correlate with severity of hepatic injury
c. Glutathione levels in the liver are increased
d. Aminotransferase levels are normal
e. N-Acetylcysteine increases renal excretion of acetaminophen

343. Which feature is characteristic of chronic hepatitis due to HBV?

a. It is more likely to occur if infection occurs in adults.
b. Seroconversion from HBeAg positive to HBeAg negative after 4 months of interferon-α therapy is 40%
c. Long-term therapy with steroids is also effective
d. The likelihood of responding to interferon is greater in patients with high levels of HBV DNA

344. The most sensitive indicator of infection with hepatitis C virus (HCV) is

a. Anti-HCV, first-generation assay against C100-3
b. Anti-HCV, second-generation assay against C200 and C22-3
c. Anti-HCV, third-generation assay against C200, C22-3, and NS5
d. Antienvelope proteins E2/NS1
e. HCV RNA

345. Which of the hepatitis viruses most commonly progresses to chronic infection and chronic hepatitis?

a. HAV
b. HBV
c. HCV
d. HEV
e. HGV

346. The clinical symptoms, signs, and outcomes following acute liver injury associated with viral hepatitis are as a consequence of the

a. Virus directly cytopathic for liver cells (hepatocytes)
b. Virus directly cytopathic to lymphoid cells in the liver
c. Immunologic response of the host (the person infected), involving cytolytic T cells
d. Primary action of viral polymerase on hepatocytes
e. Virus antibody acting on hepatocytes and lymphoid cells

347. A 30-year-old man comes to your office with complaints of fatigue, anorexia, nausea, and vomiting. He does not have fever. His urine is dark. On physical examination, his liver is slightly enlarged and minimally tender. He does not have edema or spider angiomata. Laboratory tests show the following: negative HBsAg, negative IgM anti-HAV, positive IgM anti-HBc, and negative anti-HCV. The most likely diagnosis is

a. Acute hepatitis A
b. Acute hepatitis B
c. Acute hepatitis A and B
d. Chronic hepatitis B
e. Acute hepatitis C

348. A 35-year-old woman comes to your office with complaints of fatigue, anorexia, nausea, and vomiting. She does not have fever. Her urine is dark and her stool is clay colored. On physical examination, her liver is slightly enlarged and minimally tender. She does not have edema or spider angiomata. Laboratory tests show the following: negative HBsAg, positive IgM anti-HAV, positive IgM anti-HBc, and negative anti-HCV. The most likely diagnosis is

a. Acute hepatitis A
b. Acute hepatitis B
c. Acute hepatitis A and B
d. Chronic hepatitis B
e. Acute hepatitis C

349. The most common cause of portal hypertension is

a. Hepatic vein thrombosis
b. Hepatic venoocclusive disease
c. Noncirrhotic portal fibrosis
d. Portal vein obstruction
e. Cirrhosis

350. Ascites forms in patients with cirrhosis when

a. Portal hypertension alone is present
b. Hepatic lymph flow is decreased
c. Hypoalbuminemia alone is present
d. Portal hypertension and hypoalbuminemia are present
e. Hepatic lymph flow and aldosterone secretion are decreased

351. Which is the most common precipitating event of hepatic encephalopathy?

a. Constipation
b. Hyperkalemia
c. Gastrointestinal bleeding
d. Hypernatremia
e. Acidosis

352. A serum–ascitic fluid albumin gradient of more than 1.1 g/dL is consistent with ascites caused by

a. Tuberculosis
b. Peritoneal metastases
c. Cirrhosis of the liver
d. Trauma

353. Which one of the following disorders of bilirubin metabolism shows increased unconjugated bilirubin, normal conjugated bilirubin, and lack of bilirubin in the urine?

a. Neonatal jaundice
b. Crigler-Najjar syndrome, types I and II
c. Hepatitis
d. Partial extrahepatic obstruction
e. Intravascular and extravascular hemolysis

354. Which one of the following disorders of bilirubin metabolism shows increased unconjugated bilirubin, increased conjugated bilirubin, and positive bilirubin in the urine?

a. Neonatal jaundice
b. Crigler-Najjar syndrome, types I and II
c. Hepatitis
d. Gilbert's syndrome
e. Ineffective erythropoiesis

355. In the treatment of persons with hepatic encephalopathy, which one of the following acts decreases ammonia absorption?

a. Sucrose
b. Lactulose
c. Protein
d. Glucose
e. Galactose

356. Which one of these drugs is of proven benefit in the treatment of persons with hepatic encephalopathy?

a. Levodopa
b. Bromocriptine
c. Keto analogues of essential amino acids
d. Branched-chain amino acids
e. Tetracycline

357. In spontaneous bacterial peritonitis (SBP) typically

a. Pneumococcus or other gram-positive bacteria commonly cause this infection
b. Ascitic fluid usually has a high concentration of albumin
c. Persons with normal livers and persons with advanced liver disease are equally likely to develop SBP
d. As many as 70% of patients will experience at least one recurrence within 1 year of the first episode
e. The leukocyte count in ascitic fluid is usually low, less than 100 cells/μL

358. In the hepatorenal syndrome typically

a. Urinary sodium is greater than 5 mmol/L
b. A precipitating factor occurs infrequently
c. Azotemia, hyponatremia, progressive oliguria, and hypotension are usually present
d. The urinary sediment contains a high concentration of RBC casts
e. The leukocyte count in ascitic fluid is usually low, less than 100 cells/μL

359. Chronic infection with which virus is a risk factor for the development of hepatocellular carcinoma?

a. HAV
b. HBV
c. HDV
d. HEV
e. HGV

360. Which disease is a major risk factor for development of hepatocellular carcinoma?

a. Alcoholism
b. Coombs' positive hemolytic anemia
c. Cholelithiasis
d. Cirrhosis
e. Amyloidosis

361. Which protein synthesized by the liver is commonly and significantly elevated in hepatocellular carcinoma?

a. Albumin
b. α-Fetoprotein
c. Thyroxine-binding globulin
d. Protein C
e. C-reactive protein

362. A 21-year-old college student and varsity football player comes to the emergency room with complaints of nausea, fatigue, mild right upper quadrant pain, and anorexia of several days. He has been at practice with the football team this spring and summer at a substitute practice field near the campus and he drank from a faucet of cold water at the edge of the field and near a farm. He does not use drugs. He drinks an occasional beer. Two other team members were examined recently for similar symptoms. On examination, his liver is minimally enlarged and tender. His serum bilirubin is 2.5 mg/dL and his AST and ALT are elevated. Which disease is he likely to have?

a. Cirrhosis
b. Wilson's disease
c. Hepatitis due to HAV
d. Hepatitis due to HBV
e. Hepatitis due to HCV

363. A 31-year-old man with HIV comes to your office because of nausea, fatigue, mild right upper quadrant pain, and anorexia of 3 weeks' duration. He uses intravenous illicit drugs and does so regularly. However, he previously received three doses of hepatitis B vaccine on the appropriate schedule, and he regularly takes his three-drug regimen for the treatment of his HIV. He drinks alcohol to excess, mainly for the past 2 years. On examination, he is slightly icteric and his liver is minimally enlarged and tender. His serum bilirubin is 3.0 mg/dL and his AST and ALT are significantly elevated. Which disease does he likely have?

a. Cirrhosis
b. Wilson's disease
c. Hepatitis due to HAV
d. Hepatitis due to HBV
e. Hepatitis due to HCV

364. Which hepatitis virus is transmitted almost exclusively by the fecal-oral route?

a. HAV
b. HBV
c. HCV
d. HDV   .
e. HGV

365. Primary biliary cirrhosis (PBC) typically

a. Is characterized by a circulating IgG antimitochondrial antibody present in more than 90% of patients
b. Occurs predominantly (90%) in men between the ages of 50 and 70 years with symptomatic disease
c. Can be effectively treated with glucocorticoids
d. Occurs rarely with pruritus
e. Have normal serum lipids

366. Hepatocellular adenomas

a. Have multiple hepatocellular adenomas associated with glycogen storage disease type I
b. Are mostly malignant
c. Do not have hormones playing a role in their pathogenesis
d. Occur predominantly in the left lobe of the liver
e. Occur predominantly in men

Liver Disease

Answers

327. The answer is a. *(Fauci, 14/e, pp 1664–1665.)* Alkaline phosphatase originates from bone, liver, intestine, and placenta. Elevated levels of alkaline phosphatase occur in persons with parenchymal liver diseases (slight to moderate increases in many of these cases). Impaired biliary function also shows elevated levels of alkaline phosphatase in the absence of bone disease and pregnancy. Alkaline phosphatase is not increased in diseases of the salivary glands, spleen, heart, or bladder.

328. The answer is c. *(Fauci, 14/e, pp 1664–1665.)* In parenchymal liver disease, serum albumin decreases. Albumin is synthesized in the liver and it has a half-life of 14 to 20 days. In moderate to severe parenchymal disease, the serum level of albumin decreases moderately to significantly. AST, alkaline phosphatase, prothrombin time, and GGT all increase in parenchymal liver disease.

329. The answer is c. *(Fauci, 14/e, pp 1664–1665.)* In obstructive liver disease, unlike parenchymal liver disease, the albumin level remains normal. Unlike albumin, the AST, alkaline phosphatase, prothrombin time, and GGT all increase slightly or significantly in obstructive liver disease. Of these enzymes, 5′-nucleotidase increases more in obstructive liver disease than in parenchymal liver disease.

330. The answer is b. *(Fauci, 14/e, p 1664.)* The aminotransferase ALT is found primarily in the liver. AST is found in many tissues. They are indicators of hepatocellular damage. In the hepatocyte, ALT is located only in the cytosol. Because AST occurs in many tissues, it is less specific than ALT for hepatocellular damage.

331. The answer is d. *(Fauci, 14/e, pp 1707–1709, 1666.)* The signs and symptoms in this patient suggest primary biliary cirrhosis (PBC), especially pruritus, a disease that occurs predominantly in women ages 35 to 60. The slightly elevated bilirubin and the elevated alkaline phosphatase are common in cirrhosis, and in particular, elevated alkaline phosphatase occurs in

PBC. However, a positive IgG antimitochondrial antibody is detected in more than 90% of patients with PBC and provides an important diagnostic finding.

332. The answer is c. *(Fauci, 14/e, p 1684.)* Hepatitis A virus (HAV) is transmitted solely by the fecal-oral route. Person-to-person spread of HAV is enhanced by poor personal hygiene and overcrowding. Large outbreaks, as well as sporadic cases, have been traced to consuming contaminated food, water, milk, and shellfish. Intrafamily and institutional spread are common also. It is not spread by blood transfusion and sexual contact.

333. The answer is b. *(Fauci, 14/e, p 1679.)* HBV is a DNA belonging to the Hepadnaviridae. It possesses partially single-stranded and partially double-stranded DNA and a double-shelled virion. Its major antigens are HBsAg, a surface protein, and HBcAg and HBeAg, both core proteins. The other hepatitis viruses are RNA viruses belonging to different genera and species.

334. The answer is c. *(Fauci, 14/e, pp 1680, 1688.)* Anti-HBs is the protective antibody in hepatitis B virus infection. Persons with anti-HBs are protected against reinfection with the virus. None of the other antibodies are protective. However, anti-HBe and HBC are commonly measured to gauge the progress of the infection or determine the status of a patient with a viral hepatitis.

335. The answer is d. *(Fauci, 14/e, p 1688.)* The positive HBsAg in hepatitis B virus infection, together with low levels of IgG anti-HBc, positive HBeAg, and negative anti-HBe, fit the picture of chronic HBV infection with high infectivity. In chronic or late-acute HBV of low infectivity, the HBeAg would be negative. Persons immunized with HBV vaccine show only anti-HBs. Persons who have recovered from HBV infection are negative for HBsAg.

336. The answer is c. *(Fauci, 14/e, p 1688.)* The serologic pattern in this case is a person who has recovered from HBV infection. They possess anti-HBs, the protective antibody in HBV infection, IgG anti-HBc, and anti-HBc. The anti-HBc may be positive or negative in persons who recover from HBV.

337. The answer is b. (*Fauci, 14/e, p 1689.*) Hepatitis B virus accounts for more than 50% of fulminant hepatitis cases. Also, many fulminant hepatitis cases are associated with hepatitis D virus (HDV) infection. The other hepatitis viruses are not associated with fulminant hepatitis.

338. The answer is b. (*Fauci, 14/e, p 1705.*) Mallory bodies are clumps of perinuclear, deeply eosinophilic material, or alcoholic hyaline. Their presence in hepatocytes strongly suggests alcoholic hepatitis. Similar material can be seen in hepatocytes in Wilson's disease, morbid obesity, and diabetes mellitus, but not viral hepatitis, biliary cirrhosis, or alcoholic fatty liver, or cirrhosis.

339. The answer is d. (*Fauci, 14/e, pp 1719, 2166–2168, 2174, 2179–2180.*) This patient's clinical and laboratory findings suggest Wilson's disease. These patients manifest neurologic findings, including tremors, spasticity, drooling, and dysphagia. The Babinski response may be present. The eyes show deposits of copper in Descemet's membrane of the cornea; the lack of them excludes the diagnosis. Also, the ceruloplasmin level is less than 200 mg/L.

340. The answer is d. (*Fauci, 14/e, pp 1719, 2149, 2166–2168, 2174, 2179–2180.*) Wilson's disease is an inherited copper metabolism disorder that leads to accumulation of copper in the liver, brain, and other organs. Gaucher's disease is a lipid storage disorder with a deficiency in the enzyme acid β-glucosidase. Type III glycogen storage disease is a defect in the branching enzyme. Hemochromatosis is an iron storage disorder.

341. The answer is a. (*Fauci, pp 1719, 2149, 2166–2168, 2174, 2179–2180.*) Hemochromatosis is an autosomal recessive disorder of iron storage, with impaired function of the liver. Wilson's disease is an inherited copper metabolism disorder that leads to accumulation of copper in the liver, brain, and other organs. Gaucher's disease is a lipid storage disorder with a deficiency in the enzyme acid β-glucosidase. Type III glycogen storage disease is a defect in the branching enzyme.

342. The answer is a. (*Fauci, 14/e, p 1694.*) Acetaminophen causes severe hepatic necrosis when ingested in large amounts in suicide attempts and accidentally by children. Fatal fulminant disease is usually, but not invariably, associated with ingestion of 25 g or more of the drug. Therapy should begin within 8 h of ingestion but may be effective when given as late as 24 to 36 h after the overdose. *N*-Acetylcysteine appears to act by providing a reservoir of sulfhydryl groups to bind to toxic metabolites or by stimulating synthesis and repletion of hepatic glutathione.

343. The answer is a. *(Fauci, 14/e, pp 1698–1699.)* The likelihood of chronicity after acute HBV infection varies as a function of age. Infection at birth is associated with a 90% chance of chronic infection; infection in young adulthood in immunocompetent persons is associated with an approximately 1% risk of chronicity. The likelihood of responding to interferon is greater in patients with moderate to low levels of HBV DNA and in patients with substantial elevations of aminotransferase activity. In patients with HBV, long-term therapy with glucocorticoids is ineffective and detrimental.

344. The answer is e. *(Fauci, 14/e, pp 1681–1682, 1700–1701.)* The most sensitive indicator of HCV infection is measurement of HCV RNA. The antibodies to HCV do not provide a certain measure of infection because they do not identify all persons infected with the virus.

345. The answer is c. *(Fauci, 14/e, p 1684.)* HCV progresses to chronic infection commonly. About 50 to 70% of persons infected develop chronic hepatitis. About 80 to 90% develop chronic infection. HBV progresses to chronic infection in children and adults in less than 10% of cases; however, neonates do so commonly. HAV and HEV do not progress to chronic infection.

346. The answer is c. *(Fauci, 14/e, p 1683.)* In viral hepatitis, the liver injury is due to the immunologic response of the host—the person infected. Hepatitis viruses are not directly cytopathic for hepatocytes or lymphoid cells in the liver. The viral polymerase and virus antibody acting on the hepatocytes do not play a role in liver injury in viral hepatitis.

347. The answer is b. *(Fauci, 14/e, p 1688.)* In this case, the patient has acute HBV infection signaled by the positive IgM anti-HBC. Because the HBsAg is negative, it likely is below the threshold for detection. The IgM response reflects recent infection. This serologic pattern does not fit with infection with any of the other hepatitis viruses. The symptoms and signs, lack of fever, and minimal abnormal findings on examination of the liver are consistent with the diagnosis of acute HBV.

348. The answer is c. *(Fauci, 14/e, p 1688.)* This patient has both hepatitis A and B virus infections. Both viruses can infect the same person. Clinical findings are consistent with an acute hepatitis; they are not specific for one virus. The positive IgM anti-HAV and the positive IgM anti-HBC are evidence of acute infection with both viruses. The negative HBsAg is consistent with this antigen being below the threshold of detection.

349. The answer is e. *(Fauci, 14/e, p 1710.)* The most common cause of portal hypertension is cirrhosis. About 60% of persons with cirrhosis have portal hypertension. Portal vein obstruction is the second most common cause of portal hypertension. The other diseases cause portal hypertension much less often than cirrhosis and portal vein obstruction.

350. The answer is d. *(Fauci, 14/e, p 1713.)* Ascites forms in persons with cirrhosis who suffer from both portal hypertension and hypoalbuminemia. Hepatic lymph flow is increased in cirrhosis and contributes to the ascites. Aldosterone secretion also increases ascites.

351. The answer is c. *(Fauci, 14/e, p 1715.)* Gastrointestinal bleeding is the single most important precipitating event of hepatic encephalopathy. It leads an increase in ammonia and other nitrogenous substances that are absorbed. Other factors that can precipitate hepatic encephalopathy include hyperkalemia, hypernatremia, and constipation; however, constipation is a much less important precipitating event than gastrointestinal bleeding.

352. The answer is c. *(Fauci, 14/e, p 1713.)* The serum–ascites albumin gradient provides a better classification than total protein count or other parameters. Ascites accompanying cirrhosis of the liver typically has a high serum–ascites albumin gradient (greater than 1.1 g/dL), reflecting indirectly the abnormally high hydrostatic pressure gradient between the portal bed and the ascitic compartment.

353. The answer is e. *(Fauci, 14/e, p 1676.)* This pattern of bilirubin in icterus is consistent with intravascular and extravascular hemolysis. In this condition, bilirubin turnover is increased. In partial hepatic obstruction and hepatitis, the conjugated bilirubin is increased, and in Crigler-Najjar syndrome and neonatal jaundice, the conjugated bilirubin is low.

354. The answer is c. *(Fauci, 14/e, p 1676.)* This case shows the laboratory findings in hepatitis. In Crigler-Najjar syndrome and neonatal jaundice, the conjugated bilirubin is low and no bilirubin is found in the urine. In Gilbert's syndrome and ineffective erythropoiesis, the conjugated bilirubin is low and normal, respectively, and no bilirubin is found in the urine.

355. The answer is b. *(Fauci, 14/e, p 1716.)* Lactulose, a nonabsorbable disaccharide, acts as an osmotic laxative. It works to decrease ammonia absorption. The other sugars and protein are not indicated in the treatment of hepatic encephalopathy.

356. The answer is e. *(Fauci, 14/e, p 1716.)* In addition to lactulose, antibiotics decrease ammonia production by intestinal bacteria. Tetracycline is effective, as is ampicillin and metronidazole. Neomycin is effective, but it is absorbed some and can cause renal toxicity. The role of the other drugs in the treatment of hepatic encephalopathy is unproven.

357. The answer is d. *(Fauci, 14/e, pp 1714–1715.)* Patients with cirrhosis and ascites develop SBP without any obvious primary source of infection. The ascitic fluid in these patients typically has a low concentration of albumin. An ascitic fluid count of more than 250 polymorphonuclear cells is suggestive of SBP. Empirical therapy with cefotaxime should be initiated when the diagnosis is first suspected, because enteric gram-negative bacteria are found in most cases. Recurrent episodes are relatively common; as many as 70% of the patients will experience at least one recurrence within 1 year of the first episode.

358. The answer is c. *(Fauci, 14/e, pp 1714–1715.)* Worsening azotemia, hyponatremia, progressive oliguria, and hypotension signal the hepatorenal syndrome. It may be precipitated by severe GI bleeding, sepsis, or overly vigorous attempts at diuresis. Also, it may occur without any obvious cause. Typically, the urine sodium concentration is less than 5 mmol/L. The urinary sediment is unremarkable.

359. The answer is b. *(Fauci, 14/e, pp 578–579.)* HBV is a clear risk factor for development of hepatocellular carcinoma. HCV also is a risk factor for hepatocellular carcinoma. Except for HBV and HCV, the other hepatitis viruses apparently play no role as risk factors in this carcinoma.

360. The answer is d. *(Fauci, 14/e, pp 578–579.)* Cirrhosis is a major risk factor for development of hepatocellular carcinoma. The risk of hepatocellular carcinoma in a cirrhotic liver is about 3% a year. The other diseases play no role.

361. The answer is b. *(Fauci, 14/e, p 579.)* α-Fetoprotein levels greater than 500 μg/L are found in about 70 to 80% of patients with hepatocellular carcinoma. The other proteins are synthesized in the liver but do not increase in carcinoma of the liver. Persistence of high levels of α-fetoprotein over 500 to 1000 μg/L in an adult with liver disease and without an obvious gastrointestinal cancer should be investigated for hepatocellular carcinoma.

362. The answer is c. *(Fauci, 14/e, pp 1684.)* In this case, the likelihood is that the college student drank contaminated water. The clinical and laboratory findings fit hepatitis due to HAV. He drinks too little and for too few years to have cirrhosis. HBV and HCV are parenterally spread and he has no evidence of that. Wilson's disease is an inherited disorder of copper metabolism for which this patient has no findings.

363. The answer is e. *(Fauci, 14/e, pp 1684.)* Hepatitis C virus occurs in persons with HIV and it is transmitted parenterally. The clinical and laboratory findings are consistent with this diagnosis. His heavy drinking is for too short a time for cirrhosis to develop, although he might have fat deposits in the liver. He had received HBV vaccine, thus protecting him from this infection.

364. The answer is a. *(Fauci, 14/e, pp 1684.)* HAV is transmitted exclusively by the fecal-oral route. The other hepatitis viruses, HBV, HCV, HDV, and HGV, are transmitted parenterally.

365. The answer is a. *(Fauci, 14/e, pp 1707–1708.)* The cause of PBC remains unknown. A circulating IgG antimitochondrial antibody is detected in more than 90% of the cases. Among patients with symptomatic disease, 90% are women between the ages of 35 and 60 years. In the treatment of PBC, glucocorticoids are ineffective and may actually worsen the bone disease.

366. The answer is a. *(Fauci, 14/e, p 578.)* Hepatocellular adenomas are benign tumors that occur predominantly in women and are influenced by hormones, mainly oral contraceptives. They occur mostly in the right lobe of the liver. Multiple adenomas in the liver have been associated with glycogen storage disease type I.

Thyroid and Pituitary Disorders

Questions

DIRECTIONS: Each item below contains a question or incomplete statement followed by suggested responses. Select the **one best** response to each question.

367. In a patient with iodine-deficiency goiter who moves from an iodine-deficient area to an iodine-replete area, the occurrence of hyperthyroidism most likely represents

a. Graves' disease
b. Jod-Basedow phenomenon
c. Choriocarcinoma
d. Struma ovarii
e. Toxic multinodular goiter

368. Thyrotoxicosis and uniformly increased radioactive iodine uptake in the thyroid can occur without any thyrotropin receptor antibodies or any thyroid autoimmunity in

a. Graves' disease
b. Jod-Basedow phenomenon
c. Choriocarcinoma
d. Struma ovarii
e. Toxic multinodular goiter

369. Pretibial myxedema is associated with

a. Graves' disease
b. Jod-Basedow phenomenon
c. Choriocarcinoma
d. Struma ovarii
e. Toxic multinodular goiter

370. Infiltration of orbital soft tissue and extraocular muscles with lymphocytes, mucopolysaccharides, and fluid is seen with

a. Graves' disease
b. Jod-Basedow phenomenon
c. Choriocarcinoma
d. Struma ovarii
e. Toxic multinodular goiter

371. Thyrotoxicosis with a low uptake of iodine in the thyroid bed but uptake in the pelvis can be seen with

a. Graves' disease
b. Jod-Basedow phenomenon
c. Choriocarcinoma
d. Struma ovarii
e. Toxic multinodular goiter

372. The most common cause of spontaneous hypothyroidism in the U.S. is

a. Iodine deficiency
b. Lithium
c. Hashimoto's thyroiditis
d. Propylthiouracil
e. Toxic multinodular goiter

373. The most common cause of goiter in developing nations is

a. Iodine deficiency
b. Lithium
c. Hashimoto's thyroiditis
d. Propylthiouracil
e. Toxic multinodular goiter

374. Endemic goiter results from

a. Iodine deficiency
b. Lithium
c. Hashimoto's thyroiditis
d. Propylthiouracil
e. Toxic multinodular goiter

375. The conversion of T_4 to T_3 is inhibited by

a. Iodine deficiency
b. Lithium
c. Hashimoto's thyroiditis
d. Propylthiouracil
e. Toxic multinodular goiter

376. High levels of thyroidal peroxidase antibody are found with

a. Iodine deficiency
b. Lithium
c. Hashimoto's thyroiditis
d. Propylthiouracil
e. Toxic multinodular goiter

377. A patient without symptoms and without a recent illness is found to have a normal free T_4 and elevated TSH which are confirmed on repeated measurements. The most likely explanation is

a. Hyperthyroidism
b. Nonthyroidal illness (sick euthyroidism)
c. Estrogen therapy
d. Subclinical hypothyroidism
e. Familial (euthyroid) dysalbuminenic hyperthyroxinemia

378. The pattern of normal TSH, normal T_4, and low T_3 is most consistent with

a. Hyperthyroidism
b. Nonthyroidal illness (sick euthyroidism)
c. Estrogen therapy
d. Subclinical hypothyroidism
e. Familial (euthyroid) dysalbuminenic hyperthyroxinemia

379. A low TSH, high T_4, and high T_3 suggests

a. Hyperthyroidism
b. Nonthyroidal illness (sick euthyroidism)
c. Estrogen therapy
d. Subclinical hypothyroidism
e. Familial (euthyroid) dysalbuminenic hyperthyroxinemia

380. The pattern of normal TSH, high T_4, and high T_3 is seen often with

a. Hyperthyroidism
b. Nonthyroidal illness (sick euthyroidism)
c. Estrogen therapy
d. Subclinical hypothyroidism
e. Familial (euthyroid) dysalbuminenic hyperthyroxinemia

381. A patient with a low TSH and high T_3 most likely has

a. Hyperthyroidism
b. Nonthyroidal illness (sick euthyroidism)
c. Estrogen therapy
d. Subclinical hypothyroidism
e. Familial (euthyroid) dysalbuminenic hyperthyroxinemia

382. The most common variety of thyroid cancer is

a. Thyroid lymphoma
b. Medullary thyroid carcinoma
c. Papillary thyroid carcinoma
d. Anaplastic thyroid carcinoma
e. Follicular thyroid carcinoma

383. A patient with thyroid cancer is told that he has a life expectancy of less than 6 months from diagnosis. The variety of thyroid cancer with this prognosis is

a. Thyroid lymphoma
b. Medullary thyroid carcinoma
c. Papillary thyroid carcinoma
d. Anaplastic thyroid carcinoma
e. Follicular thyroid carcinoma

384. A patient with chronic autoimmune (Hashimoto's) thyroiditis develops a rapidly enlarging thyroid mass. Most likely this is

a. Thyroid lymphoma
b. Medullary thyroid carcinoma
c. Papillary thyroid carcinoma
d. Anaplastic thyroid carcinoma
e. Follicular thyroid carcinoma

385. Psammoma bodies are a histologic feature of

a. Thyroid lymphoma
b. Medullary thyroid carcinoma
c. Papillary thyroid carcinoma
d. Anaplastic thyroid carcinoma
e. Follicular thyroid carcinoma

386. Elevated plasma calcitonin is seen with

a. Thyroid lymphoma
b. Medullary thyroid carcinoma
c. Papillary thyroid carcinoma
d. Anaplastic thyroid carcinoma
e. Follicular thyroid carcinoma

387. A 40-year-old patient with a recent viral infection presents with a significantly tender gland, low radioiodine uptake, and signs and symptoms of thyrotoxicosis. This presentation is most likely

a. Graves' disease
b. Subacute thyroiditis
c. Toxic multinodular goiter
d. Hashimoto's thyroiditis
e. Toxic adenoma

388. A 65-year-old man presents with signs and symptoms of thyrotoxicosis. His radioiodine scan and 24-h uptake show a patchy pattern but normal amount of radioiodine uptake. This presentation is most consistent with

a. Graves' disease
b. Subacute thyroiditis
c. Toxic multinodular goiter
d. Hashimoto's thyroiditis
e. Toxic adenoma

389. A 30-year-old woman with thyrotoxicosis has a diffusely enlarged gland on palpation of the neck. Her thyroid scan and 24-h uptake show uniformity of uptake and an increased percentage uptake. This patient has

a. Graves' disease
b. Subacute thyroiditis
c. Toxic multinodular goiter
d. Hashimoto's thyroiditis
e. Toxic adenoma

390. A 45-year-old man presents for frontal bossing and enlarged nose, tongue, and jaw. He has doughy palms and spadelike fingers. The best screening test to establish the diagnosis is

a. Random growth hormone
b. Insulin-like growth factor type 1 (IGF-1)
c. TSH
d. Prolactin
e. Fasting blood sugar

391. On the basis of physical findings, you suspect a 48-year-old woman has acromegaly. The definitive diagnostic test for acromegaly is measurement of growth hormone in which of the following settings?

a. Random
b. TRH stimulation test
c. Insulin tolerance test
d. Oral glucose tolerance test
e. LHRH stimulation test

392. You confirm acromegaly in a 58-year-old woman, and a MRI of the pituitary shows a microadenoma. The best choice for treatment is

a. Transsphenoidal surgery
b. Medical therapy with somatostatin agonist
c. Irradiation
d. Medical therapy with bromocriptine
e. Transfrontal surgery

393. Untreated acromegaly results in decreased life expectancy from

a. Prognathism
b. Renal hypertrophy
c. Skin tags
d. Colon carcinoma
e. Cervical arthropathy

394. A 30-year-old woman presents with a 6-month history of amenorrhea. Your initial evaluation should include measurement of

a. Prolactin
b. Estradiol
c. Progesterone
d. Testosterone
e. DHEA-S

395. A 28-year-old woman develops galactorrhea without amenorrhea. Your evaluation should include

a. Estradiol
b. Progesterone
c. Prolactin
d. Testosterone
e. DHEA-S

396. A 47-year-old man presents with headache, impotence, and galactorrhea for the past 2 months. A likely hormonal profile on this patient would be

a. Low testosterone, high LH, and low prolactin
b. Low testosterone, low LH, and low prolactin
c. Low testosterone, high LH, and high prolactin
d. Normal testosterone, normal LH, and normal prolactin
e. Low testosterone, low LH, and high prolactin

397. A 28-year-old woman presents with amenorrhea and galactorrhea, after beginning a new medication recently. The most likely medication is

a. Haloperidol
b. Lisinopril
c. Fluoxetine
d. Amitriptyline
e. Buspirone

398. A 25-year-old woman presents with amenorrhea and galactorrhea. Thyroid function tests are normal. The prolactin level is 350 μg/L (normal is less than 20). The most likely cause for her hyperprolactinemia is

a. Microadenoma
b. Macroadenoma
c. Antidepressant use
d. Exercise induced
e. Antihypertensive therapy

399. A 26-year-old woman has been amenorrheic for 2.5 months. Your first choice for diagnostic evaluation is

a. hCG
b. LH
c. Estradiol
d. Prolactin
e. Progesterone

400. A 40-year-old man has erectile dysfunction. He is noted to have hyperprolactinemia (prolactin of 400 μg/L). On MRI a macroadenoma with supersellar extension is found. The best course of therapy for the patient is

a. Medical therapy with bromocriptine
b. Transsphenoidal surgery
c. Transfrontal surgery
d. Medical therapy with somatostatin agonist
e. Thyroxine

401. A 35-year-old man has a prolactinoma and a history of severe peptic ulcer disease. There is a family history of pituitary tumors. The findings of what other diagnostic test at this time may be abnormal and potentially useful in diagnosis?

a. Fasting blood sugar
b. Serum calcium
c. Serum calcitonin
d. Urinary metanephrine
e. Serum ferritin

402. A 45-year-man has decreased libido and decreased sexual function. A large pituitary tumor is found. His prolactin is 20 (less than 15). Testing of his pituitary-gonadal axis most likely will show

a. Normal testosterone and low LH
b. High testosterone and normal LH
c. Low testosterone and low LH
d. Normal testosterone and normal LH
e. Low testosterone and high LH

403. A 16-year-old boy presents without pubertal development or development of secondary sexual characteristics. He cannot smell (anosmia). The baseline testosterone and the LH response to LHRH most likely are

a. Low testosterone and normal LHRH response
b. Normal testosterone and normal LHRH response
c. High testosterone and normal LHRH response
d. Low testosterone and no LHRH response
e. Low testosterone and exaggerated LHRH response

404. A 58-year-old woman presents as an outpatient with lethargy, fatigue, and cold intolerance. Thyroid function testing reveals a free T_4 of 0.5 (0.7 to 2.0) and a TSH of 0.1 (0.5 to 5). The best next diagnostic test is

a. Thyroid scan and uptake
b. MRI of the pituitary
c. Prolactin
d. Thyroid autoantibodies
e. T_3

405. A 59-year-old man presents with heat intolerance and tremor. Thyroid function testing reveals a free T_4 of 3.0 (0.7 to 2.0) and TSH of 6.0 (0.5 to 5). The next best diagnostic test is

a. Thyroid scan and uptake
b. MRI of the pituitary
c. Prolactin
d. Thyroid autoantibodies
e. T_3

406. A 25-year-old woman presents with increasing obesity, amenorrhea, hypertension, and abdominal stria. The next best diagnostic test is

a. Prolactin
b. Free T_4 and TSH
c. Overnight dexamethasone suppression test
d. Random cortisol
e. ACTH

407. A 30-year-old man presents with weight gain, dorsocervical fat pad, and proximal muscle weakness. His urinary free cortisol is significantly elevated and does not suppress with dexamethasone. The plasma ACTH is undetectable. Your next best diagnostic test is

a. Serum antidiuretic hormone (ADH)
b. Chest CT
c. MRI of the pituitary
d. ACTH stimulation test
e. Abdominal CT

408. A 65-year-old man with a lung mass has increasing skin pigmentation and significant muscle weakness and wasting. Urinary free cortisol is 690 μg/24 h (10 to 80) and is nonsuppressible. Which of the following tests would probably be most diagnostic?

a. ACTH stimulation test
b. MRI of the pituitary
c. CT of the abdomen
d. Plasma ACTH
e. Parathyroid hormone

409. A 48-year-old woman with a history of pituitary surgery and irradiation is scheduled for elective surgery. She currently requires replacement thyroxine, hydrocortisone, estrogen, and progesterone. In the perioperative period you will treat her with

a. Glucose infusion
b. Increased hydrocortisone
c. ACTH infusion
d. Increased estrogen
e. Increased thyroxine

410. A 23-year-old woman presents with weakness and amenorrhea. She is clinically hypothyroid. A CT scan of the pituitary shows an expanded sella with a large cystic component with calcifications. The most likely diagnosis is

a. Pituitary macroadenoma
b. Empty sella syndrome
c. Craniopharyngioma
d. Optic glioma
e. Hypothalamic hamartoma

411. Patients with pituitary macroadenoma present most commonly with

a. Bitemporal hemianopsia
b. Unilateral optic atrophy
c. Left or right homonymous visual field defect
d. Unilateral center scotoma
e. Left or right superior temporal defect

412. A 45-year-old man has decreased libido and erectile dysfunction. He has noted increasing pigmentation. He has developed liver disease and arthropathy recently. The next best diagnostic test is

a. Serum TSH
b. Serum calcium
c. Serum prolactin
d. Serum ferritin
e. Serum gastrin

Thyroid and Pituitary Disorders

Answers

367. The answer is b. (*McPhee, 2e, pp 475–479.*) Thyrotoxicosis can have several etiologies. Iodine-induced hyperthyroidism is called the Jod-Basedow phenomenon and can occur in patients with endemic goiter who move to areas where iodine is plentiful.

368. The answer is c. (*McPhee, 2e, pp 475–479.*) Diffusely increased radioiodine uptake in the thyroid accompanying thyrotoxicosis usually indicates Graves' disease, in which the thyrotropin receptors are stimulated by antibodies. However, in patients with choriocarcinoma high levels of human chorionic gonadotropin can also stimulate the thyrotropin receptor and produce the same finding.

369–370. The answers are 369: a; 370: a. (*McPhee, 2e, pp 475–479.*) Graves' disease is associated with related autoimmune phenomena in other tissues such as Graves' ophthalmopathy in the orbit and pretibial myxedema in the skin.

371. The answer is d. (*McPhee, 2e, pp 475–497.*) Ovarian teratomas can contain thyroid tissue (struma ovarii) and rarely cause thyrotoxicosis with excess thyroid hormone produced by the teratoma rather than the thyroid.

372. The answer is c. (*McPhee, 2e, pp 480–486; Fauci, 14e, pp 2021–2023.*) Hypothyroidism can result from several causes including congenital defects, chronic autoimmune thyroiditis (Hashimoto's thyroiditis), medications (thionamides, lithium, iodine), other iatrogenic causes, iodine deficiency, and hypothalamic or pituitary insufficiency. Chronic autoimmune thyroiditis is the most common cause of hypothyroidism in the U.S.

373. The answer is a. (*McPhee, 2e, pp 480–486; Fauci, 14e, pp 2021–2023.*) World-wide, iodine deficiency (endemic) goiter is very common. It is not common in the United States or other countries where salt is fortified with iodine.

374. The answer is a. (*McPhee, 2e, pp 480–486; Fauci, 14e, pp 2021–2023.*) Endemic goiter is usually associated with iodine deficiency. Worldwide it is very common.

375. The answer is d. (*McPhee, 2e, pp 480–486; Fauci, 14e, pp 2021–2023.*) Propylthiouracil, propranolol, glucocorticoids, and iodine inhibit conversion of T_4 to T_3.

376. The answer is c. (*McPhee, 2e, pp 480–486; Fauci, 14e, pp 2021–2023.*) Chronic autoimmune thyroiditis (Hashimoto's thyroiditis) is the most common cause of hypothyroidism in the U.S. and it is associated with high levels of thyroid autoantibodies.

377. The answer is d. (*McPhee, 2e, pp 470–475, 485–486; Fauci, 14e, 2016–2019.*) Laboratory measurements of thyroid hormones and thyroid-stimulating hormone have proven invaluable in determining the true functional status of the thyroid gland. However, various medications and nonthyroidal illnesses can alter certain values, so usually a combination of values is used to make a diagnosis. TSH values tend to be the most reliable in the absence of hypothalamic or pituitary disease, and mild elevation is seen in hypothyroidism before free T_4 declines.

378. The answer is b. (*McPhee, 2e, pp 470–475, 485–486; Fauci, 14e, 2016–2019.*) In severe nonthyroidal illness, T_3 declines first, followed by T_4 if the disease is severe enough, but TSH is usually normal.

379. The answer is a. (*McPhee, 2e, pp 470–475, 485–486; Fauci, 14e, 2016–2019.*) Low TSH with high T_4 and T_3 or T_3 alone (T_3 toxicosis) reflects hyperthyroidism.

380. The answer is c. (*McPhee, 2e, pp 470–475, 485–486; Fauci, 14e, 2016–2019.*) Estrogens increase thyroxine-binding globulin, elevating total T_4 and T_3, whereas free T_4, free T_3, and TSH remain normal.

381. The answer is a. (*McPhee, 2e, pp 470–475, 485–486; Fauci, 14e, 2016–2019.*) Low TSH with high T_4 and T_3 or T_3 alone (T_3 toxicosis) reflects hyperthyroidism.

382. The answer is c. (*Fauci, 14e, pp 2030–2033.*) Thyroid cancers may arise from the thyroid follicular epithelium, the parafollicular C cells, or lymphoid cells in the thyroid. Papillary carcinomas, including tumors with mixed papillary and follicular elements, are most common and account for 70% of thyroid cancers. Fifteen percent of thyroid cancers have purely follicular histology.

383. The answer is d. (*Fauci, 14e, pp 2030–2033.*) The prognosis of anaplastic cancers, which likely represent dedifferentiation of better differentiated papillary or follicular carcinomas, is very poor with average survival less than 6 months.

384. The answer is a. (*Fauci, 14e, pp 2030–2033.*) Thyroid lymphomas constitute about 5% of thyroid cancers and occur most often in patients with Hashimoto's thyroiditis. Lymphomas and anaplastic carcinomas tend to grow rapidly.

385. The answer is c. (*Fauci, 14e, pp 2030–2033.*) Psammoma bodies are a feature of papillary carcinomas.

386. The answer is b. (*Fauci, 14e, pp 2030–2033.*) Medullary thyroid carcinomas secrete calcitonin, arise in the calcitonin-producing parafollicular cells, and account for about 5% of thyroid cancers.

387. The answer is b. (*Fauci, 14e, pp 2016, 2023–2030, 2033–2034.*) The pattern and amount of radioiodine uptake on ^{123}I scan is fundamental to the correct diagnosis of thyrotoxicosis. Low-uptake thyrotoxicosis can occur when there is destruction of the thyroid follicles with release of thyroid hormone, such as in subacute thyroiditis, which usually presents as an exquisitely painful gland. Iodine-induced hyperthyroidism, factitious hyperthyroidism, and painless (silent) thyroiditis also cause low-uptake thyrotoxicosis.

388. The answer is c. (*Fauci, 14e, pp 2016, 2023–2030, 2033–2034.*) Patchy radioiodine uptake is common in multinodular goiter and Hashimoto's thyroiditis, but hyperthyroidism with normal or increased uptake typifies toxic multinodular goiter.

389. The answer is a. *(Fauci, 14e, pp 2016, 2023–2030, 2033–2034.)* In Graves' disease, the uptake tends to be increased and more uniform. Uptake may be increased without thyrotoxicosis in conditions characterized by defects in organification of iodine, such as is found in some patients with Hashimoto's thyroiditis, but the uptake tends to be patchy.

390. The answer is b. *(Fauci, 14/e, p 1982.)* The best screening test for suspected acromegaly is an IGF-1. Random growth hormone varies too much to be useful. IGF-1 is more consistent and does not fluctuate episodically throughout the day. TSH and prolactin may be abnormal but are not diagnostic of acromegaly. Fasting blood sugar may be elevated in this patient, but again it is not diagnostic.

391. The answer is d. *(Fauci, 14e, p 1982.)* The most definitive and widely accepted test for the diagnosis of acromegaly is the response of growth hormone during an oral glucose tolerance test. Typically, the growth hormone at baseline in acromegaly will be greater than 5 µg/L. In normal patients, the growth hormone will suppress to less than 2 with an oral glucose tolerance test (OGTT). In patients with acromegaly the GH values may rise, show no change, or suppress partially but not less than 2. A single random growth hormone is not useful, because of the pulsatility in growth hormone. TRH does stimulate growth hormone in many patients with acromegaly, but not all. The insulin tolerance test is a stimulation test of growth hormone and not a suppression test.

392. The answer is a. *(Fauci, 14/e, p 1982.)* Transsphenoidal surgery has the advantages of potential cure with rapid therapeutic response. If the tumor is completely resected, the patient may experience a complete cure. Medical therapy with somatostatin agonist or bromocriptine is helpful, but the patient is dependent on medical therapy indefinitely. Irradiation takes years for full effectiveness and the patient may develop hypopituitarism. Transfrontal surgery is rarely used now.

393. The answer is d. *(Fauci, 14/e, p 1981.)* Patients with untreated acromegaly have shortened life expectancy and develop complications of cardiovascular, cerebrovascular, and respiratory disease. There are recent studies suggesting patients with acromegaly have increased frequency of polyps and subsequent development of colon carcinoma. Bowel surveillance has been suggested. Cervical arthropathy is a frequent complication of acromegaly but does not directly decrease life expectancy.

394. The answer is a. *(Fauci, 14/e, p 1975.)* A common presentation for hyperprolactinemia is amenorrhea. Important in the initial evaluation of amenorrhea is a prolactin determination. Estradiol and progesterone typically are not measured in initial evaluation of amenorrhea. Testosterone and DHEA-S are markers for androgen excess, which may be present in this patient, but do not need to be measured initially.

395. The answer is c. *(Fauci, 14/e, p 1975.)* Galactorrhea in young women is often associated with hyperprolactinemia. Estradiol and progesterone can be useful markers of gonadal function but do not give further diagnostic information. Similarly, testosterone and DHEA-S do not give more diagnostic information.

396. The answer is e. *(Fauci, 14/e, p 1975.)* Men frequently present with marked hyperprolactinemia from a macroadenoma. Presenting manifestations typically are sexual dysfunction and decreased libido. The prolactin causes decrease in LH and concomitant decrease in testosterone. Thus, the patient will have a high prolactin associated with a low LH and low testosterone. The pattern of low testosterone, high LH, and low prolactin is typical of primary hypergonadism.

397. The answer is a. *(Fauci, 14/e, p 1975.)* Medications are important in the differential diagnosis of hyperprolactinemia. Prolactin release is under inhibitory control primarily from dopaminergic neurons in the hypothalamus. Dopamine attaches to D_2 receptors on lactotrophs to reduce prolactin release. Dopamine antagonists reduce the inhibition. A common drug that causes increased prolactin with possible amenorrhea and galactorrhea is haloperidol, a dopamine antagonist. Lisinopril has no effect on prolactin levels. The antidepressants fluoxetine and amitriptyline and anxiolytic bupropion may cause small changes in prolactin levels but rarely enough to cause a clinical syndrome.

398. The answer is b. *(Fauci, 14/e, p 1975.)* The serum level of prolactin correlates roughly with the size of the tumor. Prolactin levels greater than

300 are most likely associated with macroadenoma. Increases in prolactin due to medications are usually less than 100. Microadenomas usually do not exceed levels of 200 to 300.

399. The answer is a. *(Fauci, 14/e, p 1975.)* The first choice in testing in this patient is a pregnancy test. If her prolactin level was measured without a pregnancy test, an elevation of prolactin could be wrongly considered primary rather than due to pregnancy. The other tests of LH, estradiol, progesterone are not first choices in the evaluation of amenorrhea.

400. The answer is a. *(Fauci, 14/e, p 1976.)* Established therapy of hyperprolactinemia from a pituitary adenoma is treatment with a dopamine agonist such as bromocriptine. Surgical therapy usually does not result in a cure in a macroadenoma and is reserved for those patients who are intolerant to dopamine agonist. Transfrontal surgery is rarely used. Somatostatin agonist and thyroxine have little effects on hyperprolactinemia.

401. The answer is b. *(Fauci, 14/e, p 1975, 2131.)* This patient may have multiple endocrine neoplasia syndrome-1, which presents with pituitary tumors, pancreatic tumors, and hyperparathyroidism. With the history of severe peptic ulcer disease (possible Zollinger-Ellison syndrome) and family history of pituitary tumors, one must suspect MEN-1. A serum calcium will be useful in diagnosing potential hyperparathyroidism. Calcitonin and urinary metanephrines are elevated and characteristic of MEN-2. Serum ferritin and fasting blood sugar would be elevated in hemochromatosis.

402. The answer is c. *(Fauci, 14/e, p 1984.)* The patient has a common presentation for secondary hypogonadism. The large tumor is inhibiting LH secretion with consequently low testosterone secretion. No other pattern fits this clinical presentation.

403. The answer is a. *(Fauci, 14/e, p 1984.)* This patient most typically has Kallmann's syndrome. This is a deficiency in the secretion of LHRH from the hypothalamus. Typically, these patients will respond to LHRH, although they may need LHRH priming. Testosterone will be low from the lack of LHRH stimulation of LH secretion.

404. The answer is b. *(Fauci, 14/e, p 1985.)* This patient presents with clinical manifestations of hypothyroidism with a low free T_4. Secondary hypothyroidism is suggested by the low TSH. The diagnostic test of choice is a MRI of the pituitary for evaluation of a possible pituitary tumor.

405. The answer is b. *(Fauci, 14/e, p 1985.)* The patient likely has pituitary TSH–induced hyperthyroidism. This is a rare diagnosis. However, the pattern of elevated free T_4 and elevated TSH is nearly diagnostic for this disorder. The next diagnostic test is a MRI of the pituitary to evaluate for the presence of microadenoma or macroadenoma.

406. The answer is c. *(Fauci, 14/e, p 1986.)* This patient presents with a high suspicion for Cushing's syndrome. The initial step in the evaluation should be an overnight dexamethasone suppression test. Failure to suppress would indicate high likelihood of Cushing's syndrome. A random cortisol is not sufficient to screen for Cushing's syndrome. An ACTH by itself is not useful.

407. The answer is e. *(Fauci, 14/e, p 1986.)* The suppression of ACTH is characteristic of adrenal adenoma or carcinoma. A CT scan will evaluate for the presence of adrenal tumor. Chest CT is useful in ectopic ACTH secretion. A MRI of the pituitary is useful in pituitary dependent Cushing's disease. The ACTH stimulation test and serum ADH are not diagnostic in this disease.

408. The answer is d. *(Fauci, 14/e, p 1986.)* This patient's presentation suggests ectopic ACTH secretion and ACTH will likely be elevated above 300. A MRI of the pituitary and CT of the abdomen are not useful, because the source of ACTH is from the small cell carcinoma in the lung mass.

409. The answer is b. *(Fauci, 14/e, p 1994.)* This patient has classic history for hypopituitarism. During surgical stress she will require increased replacement dose of steroids. The other treatments will not cover her need for increased glucocorticoids and will not be helpful.

410. The answer is c. *(Fauci, 14/e, p 1988.)* This is the common CT finding and clinical presentation for craniopharyngioma. Empty sella does not usually cause marked enlargement of the sella, and there is no cystic structure with calcification. Pituitary macroadenomas can expand the sella but are not commonly cystic and calcified. Optic glioma and hypothalamic hamartoma are rarely cystic.

411. The answer is a. *(Fauci, 14/e, p 1990.)* Classic presentation is bitemporal hemianopsia with the other visual field disturbances less common.

412. The answer is d. *(Fauci, 14/e, p 1993, 2150.)* The patient has classic manifestations of hemochromatosis that impairs hypothalamic pituitary function. Serum ferritin is potentially diagnostic in this patient. All the other tests are not diagnostic for hemochromatosis.

Reproductive System

Questions

DIRECTIONS: Each item below contains a question or incomplete statement followed by suggested responses. Select the **one best** response to each question.

413. Which of the following organs is not a major estrogen-dependent tissue in women?

a. Brain
b. Thyroid
c. Hypothalamus
d. Pituitary
e. Ovaries

414. Which of the following organs does not require androgens for proper growth in males?

a. Brain
b. Prostate
c. Epididymis
d. Vas deferens
e. Long bones

415. A patient has an excess of 17α-hydroxyprogesterone and 17α-hydroxypregnenolone in the urine, and no androgens. Which enzyme is deficient?

a. 20,22-Desmolase
b. 3β-Hydroxysteroid dehydrogenase
c. 17-Hydroxylase
d. 17,20-Desmolase (17,20 lyase)
e. 17-Ketoreductase

416. Which of these hormones is also produced in significant amounts outside of the gonads?

a. Estrone
b. Estradiol
c. Androstenedione
d. Testosterone
e. Dihydrotestosterone

417. A 22-year-old woman marathon runner comes into the office complaining of amenorrhea for 8 months. There has been no weight change, and the serum pregnancy test is negative. She has never been pregnant. Menarche was at 13 years of age, and she had monthly menses until 8 months ago. Physical exam shows a women who is 66 inches tall, 90 pounds, and is otherwise fully normal. Why does she have amenorrhea?

a. Hypothyroidism
b. Prolactinoma
c. Early menopause
d. Resistance to LH and FSH
e. Excessive exercise

418. A young couple, both in their 20s, have been trying for 2 years to have a baby. The male comes into the office and on workup has oligospermia, high LH, high FSH, and a normal karyotype. How do you treat him?

a. Do nothing
b. Testosterone injections
c. Check the partner for causes of infertility
d. Infertility counseling

419. A 28-year-old woman presents to the office with 2 days of abdominal pain and a positive pregnancy test. Her last menstrual period was 9 weeks ago. She reports no dysuria. She reports a history of two episodes of pelvic inflammatory disease. Which of these is the most likely cause of the abdominal pain?

a. Endometriosis
b. Urinary tract infection
c. Ectopic pregnancy
d. Placental abruption
e. Premenstrual syndrome

420. A 38-year-old woman comes into the office with complaints of amenorrhea for 6 months, with increased cold intolerance, loss of energy, and hair loss. Her menses were normal until this episode started, and she has also gained 22 pounds over these 6 months. Her pregnancy test is negative. Which test would you now order?

a. FSH and LH
b. Estrogen levels
c. Testosterone level
d. TSH
e. Cortisol level

421. A 29-year-old woman comes into the office after three spontaneous abortions (unplanned). All three occurred at approximately 6 weeks' gestational age. Her physical exam is normal. Which of these may be the cause?

a. Ovary
b. Thyroid gland
c. Adrenal gland
d. Pituitary gland

422. Which of these medications treats benign prostatic hyperplasia by 5α-reductase inhibition?

a. Leuprolide
b. Nafarelin
c. Flutamide
d. Megesterol
e. Finasteride

423. How does pregnancy increase the risk of diabetes mellitus?

a. Causing weight gain
b. Insulin resistance
c. Placental production of human chorionic somatomammotropin
d. Increase of maternal glucocorticoids

424. Which of these hormones blocks milk production during pregnancy?

a. Progesterone
b. Prolactin
c. Chorionic somatomammotropin
d. Thyroxine
e. Insulin

425. A 40-year-old female presents with amenorrhea and hirsutism. Which hormone is in excess in this woman with polycystic ovary syndrome?

a. Estrogen
b. Progesterone
c. FSH
d. Androgens

426. Which of these is the best therapy for preeclampsia?

a. Antihypertensive medication
b. Antiseizure medication
c. Intravenous fluids
d. Delivery of the baby
e. Anticoagulation

427. Which of these findings is the best for diagnosis of a congenital absence of the vas deferens?

a. Oligospermia
b. Azoospermia
c. Normal testosterone
d. Normal LH
e. Normal FSH

428. Which abnormality of adult testicular function (infertility) occurs with normal virilization?

a. Hemochromatosis
b. Cryptorchidism
c. Isolated gonadotropism deficiency
d. Klinefelter's syndrome
e. XX male

429. A 19-year-old woman comes to the office complaining of galactor-rhea. She has never been pregnant. Which hormone is the most likely to be responsible for this situation?

a. Prolactin
b. Estrogen
c. Progesterone
d. Thyroxine
e. Cortisol

430. A 15-year-old male comes into the office complaining about a lack of pubic hair growth. He also informs you that his voice has not yet deepened, and he has no interest in sexual activity. He is an only child. Blood drawn reveals a very high testosterone level. What is the problem?

a. Low FSH and LH
b. High FSH and LH
c. Androgen insensitivity
d. Hyperthyroidism
e. XXY karyotype

431. A 52-year-old female presents to the office with a complaint of hot flashes. You suspect menopause. Which of the findings below would confirm your diagnosis?

a. Normal androgen level
b. Normal or low estrogen level
c. Normal prolactin level
d. High FSH and LH
e. High androgen level

432. Which of the following organs does ovarian estrogen production have a stimulatory effect on?

a. Ovary
b. Brain
c. Hypothalamus
d. Pituitary
e. Vagina

433. A 19-year-old pregnant female feels tired and out of pep. Her conjunctivae are pale; laboratory tests show she has a mild normocytic, normochromic anemia with a low serum iron and an increased TIBC (transferrin iron-binding capacity). Hemoccult tests are negative. Which is the likely cause of her anemia?

a. Gastrointestinal bleeding
b. Iron or folate deficiencies
c. Autoantibodies
d. Vitamin B_{12} deficiency
e. Menstrual blood loss

434. Which of the following hormones is produced by both the ovary and uterus?

a. Inhibin
b. Activin
c. Follistatin
d. Relaxin
e. Enkephalin

435. Which of the following hormones is produced both by the theca and the kidney?

a. Inhibin
b. Relaxin
c. Renin
d. Epidermal growth factor-like
e. Transforming growth factor-β

436. A 31-year-old male presents to the office due to infertility. On history, it is revealed that he has Kartagener's syndrome. Why is he infertile?

a. Oligospermia
b. Asthenospermia
c. Absence of the vas deferens
d. Epididymal obstruction
e. Undescended testes

437. A 74-year-old male presents to the office with trouble urinating for 1 week. The force of the urinary stream is reduced, but there is no difficulty starting the stream. There is no pain. What is the problem?

a. Decreased detrusor contractility
b. Detrusor instability
c. Detrusor failure
d. Acute urinary obstruction
e. Chronic urinary obstruction

438. A 65-year-old male presents to the office with benign prostatic hypertrophy and new onset hypertension. Which one medication could you give this patient to handle both diagnoses?

a. Nafarelin
b. Flutamide
c. Finasteride
d. Megesterol
e. Prazosin

439. A 28-year-old woman presents complaining of infertility. She had a healthy child 3 years ago and has been trying to get pregnant with the child's father for the last 18 months. She does not have dysmenorrhea. Her menses occur regularly, but these show significantly less flow compared with before her pregnancy. She recalls having a curettage performed to remove placental remnants. What is the diagnosis?

a. Ovarian failure
b. Hypothyroidism
c. Asherman's syndrome
d. Endometriosis
e. Prolactinoma

440. A 28-year-old previously healthy female, with no medical history is now 28 weeks pregnant. She complains of trouble seeing, polyuria, polyphagia, and polydipsia. What is her diagnosis?

a. Gestational diabetes mellitus
b. Deep venous thrombosis
c. Urinary tract infection
d. Preeclampsia

441. A 26-year-old female is about to deliver a baby. She asks you why should she breast-feed. Beyond the obvious issue of child to mother bonding, what else must you tell her?

a. It's the correct thing to do
b. Better nutrition for the baby
c. Protect the baby from infections early in life
d. Quicker weight loss
e. Good contraception

442. Which of the following is not required for successful breast-feeding?

a. Prolactin
b. Oxytocin
c. Good maternal nutrition
d. An intact neurologic axis
e. High estrogen levels

443. Which of the following hormones in excess causes male infertility?

a. FSH
b. LH
c. Testosterone
d. Cortisol
e. Prolactin

444. How do varicoceles cause male infertility?

a. Decreasing testicular blood flow
b. Increasing testicular temperature
c. Reduction of testosterone production
d. By causing testicular atrophy

445. A 52-year-old female presents to the office with a chief complaint of postmenopausal bleeding for 2 weeks. Her menopause was 7 years ago, and until 2 weeks ago had no vaginal bleeding of any kind. She was not receiving hormonal replacement. Which of the following tests need not be ordered or performed?

a. Pap smear
b. TSH
c. Prothrombin time
d. Smear for vaginal infection
e. General blood chemistry evaluation

446. In which ovarian compartment is Müllerian-inhibiting substance produced?

a. Granulosa
b. Theca
c. Follicular fluid
d. Follicles
e. Corpus luteum

447. In which ovarian compartment is plasminogen activator produced?

a. Granulosa
b. Theca
c. Follicular fluid
d. Follicles
e. Corpus luteum

448. In which ovarian compartment is transforming growth factor-α produced?

a. Granulosa
b. Theca
c. Follicular fluid
d. Follicles
e. Corpus luteum

449. In which ovarian compartment is basic fibroblast growth factor produced?

a. Granulosa
b. Theca
c. Follicular fluid
d. Follicles
e. Corpus luteum

450. In which ovarian compartment is angiotensin II produced?

a. Granulosa
b. Theca
c. Follicular fluid
d. Follicles
e. Corpus luteum

451. During the course of an evaluation for thyroid function, your patient, a 33-year-old man who is infertile, is found to have very low levels of luteinizing hormone. The likely site of his infertility is

a. Pretesticular
b. Testicular
c. Posttesticular
d. Idiopathic

452. A 41-year-old man comes to your office with his wife because she has been unable to conceive with him. He is married for the first time. His wife has two children by her previous marriage. The patient is well with no risk factors for heart disease. As a child, he had the usual communicable diseases, including chickenpox and mumps, and as an adult he received the recommended schedule of immunizations. The likely site of his infertility is

a. Pretesticular
b. Testicular
c. Posttesticular
d. Idiopathic

453. A 31-year-old man whom you treated for alcoholic intoxication at the emergency room 2 days ago comes to your office because he wants another opinion about his infertility. He has seen other physicians for this condition. Considering his excessive alcoholic intake for the past decade, the likely site of his infertility is

a. Pretesticular
b. Testicular
c. Posttesticular
d. Idiopathic

454. A 27-year-old man who suffers seizures controlled with phenytoin comes to your office because his neurologist discovered that the patient has a low FSH level. The patient is infertile. The likely site of his infertility is

a. Pretesticular
b. Testicular
c. Posttesticular
d. Idiopathic

455. A urologist refers a 20-year-old man because of hypospadias and infertility. He has been sexually active since his early teens. Recently, he married and, despite many attempts, his wife has been unable to become pregnant. The likely site of his infertility is

a. Pretesticular
b. Testicular
c. Posttesticular
d. Idiopathic

Reproductive System

Answers

413. The answer is b. *(McPhee, 2/e, p 519.)* The thyroid gland is minimally affected by estrogens, but it may have an impact on estrogen production (still unclear). The brain, hypothalamus, pituitary, ovaries, uterine epithelium, uterine tubes, and vagina are all major estrogen-dependent tissues in women.

414. The answer is a. *(McPhee, 2/e, p 547.)* The brain's growth is not affected by androgens, although there are mental changes associated with androgens. The prostate, epididymis, vas deferens, scrotum, seminal vesicles, penis, and long bones all require androgens for proper growth and physical development.

415. The answer is d. *(McPhee, 2/e, p 545; Fauci, 14/e, pp 2036, 2100.)* 20,22-Desmolase changes cholesterol to pregnenolone. 3β-hydroxysteroid dehydrogenase changes pregnenolone to progesterone and 17α-hydroxy-pregnenolone into 17α-hydroxyprogesterone. 17-Hydroxylase changes pregnenolone and progesterone into 17α-hydroxypregnenolone and 17α-hydroxyprogesterone, respectively. 17,20-Desmolase changes 17α-hydroxypregnenolone into dehydroepiandrosterone (a weak androgen) and 17α-hydroxyprogesterone into androstenedione (a weak androgen). 17-ketoreductase changes dehydroepiandrosterone and androstenedione to androstenediol and testosterone, respectively.

416. The answer is c. *(McPhee, 2/e, pp 491, 520, 545; Fauci, 14/e, p 2036.)* Estrone and estradiol are mainly produced in the ovaries in women. Testosterone and dihydrotestosterone are mainly produced in the testes. Dihydrotestosterone is also produced in the periphery directly from testosterone. Androstenedione is the main end product of the zona reticularis of the adrenal gland, in addition to being produced in the gonads.

417. The answer is e. (*McPhee, 2/e, pp 531–535; Fauci, 14/e, pp 2105–2107.*) Hypothyroid patients tend to gain weight. Prolactin-secreting tumors (prolactinomas), being located in the pituitary, would be expected to show abnormal physical examination findings at the eyes, given that the tumor typically sits on the optic chiasma. Early menopause is unlikely in a 22-year-old. Resistance to LH and FSH would have prohibited this patient from ever having menses. This leaves excessive exercise as the only remaining plausible cause in this patient.

418. The answer is b. (*McPhee, 2/e, p 552; Fauci, 14/e, pp 2092–2097.*) This patient presents with classic testosterone deficiency, as evidenced by the low sperm count and elevated gonadotropic hormones.

419. The answer is c. (*McPhee, 2/e, pp 530, 539; Fauci, 14/e, pp 812–817.*) Pelvic inflammatory disease is a cause of tubal scarring, setting the stage for an ectopic (tubal) pregnancy. As the pregnancy grows, the tube is stretched, causing pain. Endometriosis causes pain with each menstrual cycle, which is not the case here. Urinary tract infection can cause pain, but she would be expected to have dysuria. Placental abruption occurs only after 20 weeks of pregnancy. She is clearly not premenstrual, because she is pregnant.

420. The answer is d. (*McPhee, 2/e, pp 481, 532–534; Fauci, 14/e, pp 2021–2023.*) Hypothyroidism is the cause of this patient's amenorrhea. Classic findings of hypothyroidism presented here are increased cold intolerance, loss of energy, hair loss, and weight gain. TSH is the best test for this disorder, and it would be increased in the hypothyroid patient.

421. The answer is a. (*McPhee, 2/e, p 523.*) Once the woman is pregnant, she needs to maintain a high level of progesterone in the system to sustain the fetus. The corpus luteum, sitting in the ovary, has that role, under the influence of the β-hCG produced by the placenta. If the corpus luteum cannot produce enough progesterone to get the pregnancy to the tenth week, the pregnancy is lost.

422. The answer is e. (*McPhee, 2/e, p 555; Fauci, 14/e, pp 596–598.*) Leuprolide, nafarelin, and megesterol all inhibit LH secretion and thus decrease testosterone and dihydrotestosterone levels. Flutamide and megesterol all are androgen receptor inhibitors. Finasteride blocks 5α-reductase, leading to a reduction of dihydrotestosterone and net reduction of prostate size.

423. The answer is c. *(McPhee, 2/e, p 525; Barron, 2/e, pp 63–65.)* Human chorionic somatomammotropin is a counterregulatory hormone that works to protect the fetus from hypoglycemia. The net result can be hyperglycemia and thus diabetes mellitus. Weight gain does occur in pregnancy, but insulin resistance and increased production of maternal glucocorticoids have not been proven to occur.

424. The answer is a. *(McPhee, 2/e, pp 525–526; Fauci, 14/e, pp 2115–2116.)* All of these hormones are required for proper preparation of the breast to produce milk in the postpartum period, but high levels of progesterone and estrogen during pregnancy prevent actual milk production. Milk is produced postpartum, once the levels of these two hormones drop.

425. The answer is d. *(McPhee, 2/e, pp 532–535; Fauci, 14/e, pp 2106–2107.)* In polycystic ovary disease, estrogen is usually elevated from non-ovarian sources. Progesterone levels are usually unchanged. FSH is usually low. Androgens are usually elevated and are the cause for these symptoms. These androgens are produced in the ovary as the result of elevated LH. Low FSH prevents the formation of ovarian estrogen.

426. The answer is d. *(McPhee, 2/e, pp 539–540; Barron, 2/e, pp 13–14.)* Although antihypertensive medication, antiseizure medication, intravenous fluids, and anticoagulation may all take care of parts of preeclampsia, the best therapy is to deliver the baby.

427. The answer is b. *(McPhee, 2/e, p 552; Fauci, 14/e, pp 2092–2095.)* Although all of the above may be present in patients with an absent vas deferens, azoospermia is the best choice. Oligospermia, normal testosterone, normal LH, and normal FSH may also be present in a wide variety of other causes of male infertility, alone or in combination.

428. The answer is b. *(Fauci, 14/e, p 2092.)* Cryptorchidism or failure of the testes to descend from the abdominal cavity to the scrotal sac results in failure of spermatogenesis because it cannot take place in the higher temperature of the abdominal cavity. However, virilization proceeds normally. The other conditions impair fertility and androgenization.

429. The answer is a. (*McPhee, 2/e, pp 461–462, 525–526; Fauci, 14/e, pp 2116–2117.*) Prolactin is the major stimulator of breast milk production. Overproduction of prolactin leads to galactorrhea. Estrogen, progesterone, thyroxine, and cortisol are all needed for proper breast development but play no role in actual milk production.

430. The answer is c. (*McPhee, 2/e, pp 544–548; Fauci, 14/e, pp 2088, 2091–2092.*) Androgen insensitivity can present as an inability for a male child to go into puberty. Low FSH and LH are expected to yield low testosterone levels. High FSH and LH are usually markers of end organ damage and lack of feedback of testosterone on the pituitary due to low levels. Puberty can be delayed by hypothyroidism, with FSH and LH usually appropriate to the testosterone level. XXY karyotype (Klinefelter's) often has no effect on testosterone level.

431. The answer is d. (*McPhee, 2/e, pp 527–528; Fauci, 14/e, p 2012.*) In both premenopausal and menopausal women, androgen levels may be normal or high, estrogen levels normal, and prolactin level normal. Androgen production can be in the ovary or the adrenal gland. Estrogen production is mainly in the ovary prior to menopause and in the periphery by conversion of testosterone in menopause. The amount of estrogen during menopause is a function of the patient's amount of adipose tissue. High FSH and LH are the hallmarks of a lack of adequate ovarian production of both estrogen and progesterone, the chemical markers of menopause, due to lack of negative feedback.

432. The answer is e. (*McPhee, 2/e, pp 521–522.*) The effect of estrogen on the vagina, uterus, uterine tubes, and breasts is stimulatory. The effect on the ovary is paracrine. There is a negative feedback effect on the brain, hypothalamus, and pituitary.

433. The answer is b. (*Fauci, 14/e, pp 28, 640–641.*) Iron and folate deficiencies occur in pregnancy because the fetus uses these substances in large amounts. The pregnant woman needs adequate supplements of iron and folate. Autoantibodies and vitamin B_{12} are not unique causes of iron deficiency in pregnancy. The history precludes gastrointestinal bleeding and menses as causes of this patient's blood loss.

434. The answer is d. *(McPhee, 2/e, p 516.)* Relaxin is the only hormone produced both by the ovary and uterus. Inhibin is produced in the granulosa, theca, and corpus luteum. Activin is produced in the granulosa. Follistatin is produced in follicles. Enkephalin is produced by the ovary.

435. The answer is c. *(McPhee, 2/e, pp 377, 516.)* Renin is the only hormone produced by both the theca and kidney. Inhibin is produced in the granulosa, theca, and corpus luteum. Relaxin is produced in the corpus luteum, theca, placenta, and uterus. Epidermal growth factor-like is produced in granulosa and theca. Transforming growth factor-β is produced in theca, ovarian interstitial tissue, and granulosa.

436. The answer is b. *(McPhee, 2/e, p 551; Fauci, 14/e, pp 1446, 2092.)* Kartagener's syndrome is also known as the immotile cilia syndrome. Asthenospermia or poor sperm motility is due to missing dynein arms, the basic defect of Kartagener's syndrome. Kartagener's syndrome has no effect on either sperm count or basic anatomy of the male reproductive tract.

437. The answer is a. *(McPhee, 2/e, pp 557–558; Fauci, 14/e, pp 262–265.)* Detrusor instability, decreased contractility, and failure are all part of a continuum. Decreased contractility is implied by the decreased force of the stream. Instability alone has only frequency and urgency. Failure implies an inability to urinate due to muscle failure. With acute obstruction, the patient cannot void, and there is significant pain. With chronic urinary obstruction, starting the stream is also a problem.

438. The answer is e. *(McPhee, 2/e, p 557; Fauci, 14/e, p 598.)* α-Blockers, such as prazosin, can treat both hypertension and benign prostatic hypertrophy. Nafarelin, flutamide, finasteride, and megesterol have no role in blood pressure management.

439. The answer is c. *(McPhee, 2/e, pp 531–539; Fauci, 14/e, pp 2106–2108.)* One of the least recognized causes of infertility in a female is scarring of the uterus postpartum, called Asherman's syndrome. It classically follows curettage of the uterus, such as occurred here. Women with this syndrome are infertile because an inability to implant. Ovarian failure, hypothyroidism, and prolactinoma are all eliminated because she still has scant regular menses. Endometriosis causes painful menses.

440. The answer is a. (*McPhee, 2/e, pp 432, 436, 529; Barron, 2/e, pp 74–75.*) This patient presents with the classic triad of diabetes mellitus—polyuria, polyphagia and polydipsia, in combination with visual problems, which can be a marker of diabetic retinopathy. Deep venous thrombosis, urinary tract infection, and preeclampsia are all complications of pregnancy, but none present like this.

441. The answer is c. (*McPhee, 2/e, pp 526–527.*) Although all five options sound appealing, only protection of the baby from infection is a proven benefit. This occurs through immunoglobulins (IgA) in the breast milk. Now that various formulas exist, nutrition no longer is a major reason by itself to breast-feed. Quicker weight loss is an old wives' tale. The reliability of breast-feeding as a contraceptive technique is low, at best.

442. The answer is e. (*McPhee, 2/e, pp 455–456, 526–528; Fauci, 14/e, pp 1974–1978, 2115–2116.*) Prolactin stimulates milk production. Oxytocin stimulates milk ejection. Good maternal nutrition is needed to ensure adequate nutritional content of the milk. An intact neurologic axis is needed to ensure that the sucking by the baby leads to oxytocin and prolactin secretion. High estrogen levels inhibit milk production.

443. The answer is e. (*McPhee, 2/e, pp 461–462, 549; Fauci, 14/e, p 2092.*) FSH ensures sperm production. LH ensures androgen production. Testosterone is the end product of the testes, and deficiency causes infertility. Cortisol deficiency stimulates an increase in prolactin secretion. High prolactin levels are a cause of male infertility.

444. The answer is b. (*McPhee, 2/e, pp 542, 548–549; Fauci, 14/e, p 2093.*) Varicoceles (dilation of the peritesticular pampiniform plexus of veins) increase the temperature of the scrotum, and hence the testicles, by an increase in local blood flow. Sperm production is reduced by high temperatures. Testosterone production and testicular atrophy are not caused by varicoceles.

445. The answer is e. *(McPhee, 2/e, pp 481, 538; Fauci, 14/e, 2114.)* Pap smear may detect a malignancy as the cause of the bleeding; also when uterine cancer is a consideration, as it might be in this case, an endometrial biopsy should be performed. Hypothyroidism is also a cause of post-menopausal bleeding. A bleeding disorder, as documented by an elevated prothrombin time, can explain bleeding. Vaginal infections can also cause vaginal bleeding. A general chemistry evaluation at this time is too non-specific.

446. The answer is a. *(McPhee, 2/e, p 516; Fauci, 14/e, pp 2098–2100.)* Müllerian-inhibiting substance is produced in the granulosa. Other endocrine and paracrine products of the granulosa include plasminogen activator, activin, inhibin, follicle regulatory protein, insulin-like growth factor-1, epidermal growth factor-like, platelet-derived growth factor, proopiomelanocortin, and gonadotropin surge-inhibiting factor. Some of these are produced also in other ovarian compartments, such as inhibin in the theca and corpus luteum, follicle regulatory protein in the follicular fluid and theca, and epidermal growth factor-like in the theca.

447. The answer is a. *(McPhee, 2/e, p 516; Fauci, 14/e, pp 2098–2100.)* Plasminogen activator is produced in the granulosa. Other endocrine and paracrine products of the granulosa include Müllerian-inhibiting substance, activin, inhibin, follicle regulatory protein, insulin-like growth factor-1, epidermal growth factor-like, platelet-derived growth factor, proopiomelanocortin, and gonadotropin surge-inhibiting factor. Some of these are produced also in other ovarian compartments, such as inhibin in the theca and corpus luteum, follicle regulatory protein in the follicular fluid and theca, and epidermal growth factor-like in the theca.

448. The answer is b. *(McPhee, 2/e, p 516; Fauci, 14/e, pp 2098–2100.)* Transforming growth factor-α and transforming growth factor-β, renin, inhibin, relaxin are produced in the theca. Some of these are produced also in other ovarian compartments, such as transforming growth factor-α and transforming growth factor-β in the interstitial, inhibin in the granulosa and corpus luteum, and relaxin in the corpus luteum.

449. The answer is e. *(McPhee, 2/e, p 516; Fauci, 14/e, pp 2098–2100.)* Basic fibroblast growth factor is produced in the corpus luteum. Other endocrine and paracrine products of the ovarian compartments include the following: from the granulosa: Müllerian-inhibiting substance, activin, inhibin, follicle regulatory protein, insulin-like growth factor-1, epidermal growth factor-like, platelet-derived growth factor, proopio-melanocortin, and gonadotropin surge-inhibiting factor; from the theca: transforming growth factor-α and transforming growth factor-β, renin, inhibin, and relaxin; and from the follicular fluid: luteinizing inhibitor and luteinizing stimulator, oocyte meiosis inhibitor, follicle regulatory protein, and renin.

450. The answer is c. (*McPhee, 2/e, p 516; Fauci, 14/e, pp 2098–2100.*) Angiotensin II is produced in the follicular fluid, as are luteinizing inhibitor and luteinizing stimulator, oocyte meiosis inhibitor, follicle regulatory protein, and renin. Other endocrine and paracrine products of the ovarian compartments include the following: from the granulosa: Müllerian-inhibiting substance, activin, inhibin, follicle regulatory protein, insulin-like growth factor-1, epidermal growth factor-like, platelet-derived growth factor, proopiomelanocortin, and gonadotropin surge-inhibiting factor; from the theca: transforming growth factor-α and transforming growth factor-β, renin, inhibin, and relaxin; and from the corpus luteum: basic fibroblast growth factor.

451. The answer is a. (*McPhee, 2/e, pp 548–549; Fauci, 14/e, pp 2092–2095.*) Pretesticular causes are those affecting the hormones that stimulate the testicles, such as a low LH or FSH, and include various hypothalamic-pituitary disorders including panhypopituitarism and gonadotrophin deficiency. Gonadotrophin deficiency includes isolated LH deficiency and Kallmann's syndrome. Posttesticular causes are those that affect sperm transport, and testicular causes are those with a direct effect on the testicles. Idiopathic causes represent those causes that are likely genetic and not elsewhere classified.

452. The answer is b. (*McPhee, 2/e, pp 548–549; Fauci, 14/e, pp 2092–2095.*) Mumps virus infection can directly affect the testicles, producing an orchitis, often very painful, and consequently infertility. Posttesticular causes are those that affect sperm transport, and pretesticular causes are those that affect the hormones that stimulate the testicles.

453. The answer is b. *(McPhee, 2/e, pp 548–549; Fauci, 14/e, pp 2092–2095.)* Testicular causes are those with a direct effect on the testicles. Alcohol directly affects the testicles causing atrophy with inadequate sperm production. It also causes decreased plasma testosterone. Posttesticular causes are those that affect sperm transport, and pretesticular causes are those that affect the hormones that stimulate the testicles. Idiopathic causes represent those causes that are likely genetic and not elsewhere classified.

454. The answer is a. *(McPhee, 2/e, pp 548–549; Fauci, 14/e, pp 2092–2095.)* Pretesticular causes are those that affect the hormones that stimulate the testicles, such as a low LH or FSH. Phenytoin acts by reducing FSH. Other causes of a low LH or FSH include various hypothalamic-pituitary disorders, such as panhypopituitarism and gonadotrophin deficiency, including isolated LH deficiency and Kallmann's syndrome. Posttesticular causes are those that affect sperm transport, and testicular causes are those with a direct effect on the testicles. Idiopathic causes represent those causes that are likely genetic and not elsewhere classified.

455. The answer is c. *(McPhee, 2/e, pp 548–549; Fauci, 14/e, pp 2092–2095.)* Posttesticular causes of infertility are those that affect sperm transport, such as penile anatomic defects including hypospadias and epispadias. Other posttesticular causes of infertility include genital tract infections, retrograde ejaculation, and antibodies to sperm or seminal plasma. Pretesticular causes are those that affect the hormones that stimulate the testicles, and testicular causes are those with a direct effect on the testicles. Idiopathic causes represent those causes that are likely genetic and not elsewhere classified.

Nervous System

Questions

DIRECTIONS: Each item below contains a question or incomplete statement followed by suggested responses. Select the **one best** response to each question.

456. A 35-year-old man comes to your office with a complaint of recent development of headaches that are generalized in nature. He is accompanied by his wife who recently returned from a trip. She tells you that her husband has been somewhat confused at times and clumsy. He does not confirm this, but he does report that he has been short of breath at times. On examination, he is mildly tachycardia and there is a reddish appearance to his mucous membranes, which is subtle. The only recent new medical problem identified is that the patient was in a motor vehicle accident in which he was struck in the rear end, and it left him with a sore neck. The most likely diagnosis is

a. Acquired spinal stenosis (cervical)
b. Normal pressure hydrocephalus
c. Carbon monoxide poisoning
d. Cocaine toxicity
e. Muscle tension

457. A 40-year-old man is noted to have miosis of the right eye and ipsilateral ptosis. He reports that he has noted that this side of his face is not sweating when he is working recently. The most cause of this clinical picture may be

a. Pancoast tumor
b. Brainstem CVA
c. Dissection of the carotid artery
d. Idiopathic

458. A 55-year-old male describes bilateral pain in his lower back and legs with prolonged standing while working on an assembly line. Whenever he sits down and takes a break, he gets some relief, but it recurs when he resumes his job. No other inciting events can be identified. The most likely cause of this problem is

a. Degenerative joint disease
b. Degenerative disk disease
c. Peripheral vascular disease
d. Lumbar spinal stenosis

459. An elderly woman is seen at your office with a complaint of loss of vision in her left eye, which had been transient on a couple of occasions but is now persisting. She has been seen recently at urgent care centers for multiple complaints including generalized fatigue, left-sided dull boring headaches with occasional sharp jabbing sensations, and arthritic complaint in the hips. In addition, she reports some recent loss of 7 to 10 pounds. The only remarkable finding on the routine labs obtained from her prior evaluations is an elevated alkaline phosphatase. You determine that the likely cause of her condition is

a. Glaucoma
b. Brain tumor arising anterior to the optic chiasm
c. Optic neuritis
d. Temporal arteritis

460. A middle-aged female arrives at your office after not seeing a physician for many years to have a general physical performed. Overall, she appears healthy but a poorly reacting left pupil is noted when a pen light is used. Instillation of a weak solution of pilocarpine leads to constriction of the pupil quickly. Your diagnosis is

a. Argyll Robertson pupil
b. Adie's tonic pupil
c. Trauma-induced pupil dysfunction
d. Horner's syndrome

461. In the above patient, what other abnormality on physical would be consistent with the diagnosis?

a. Ptosis
b. Decreased visual acuity on Snellen's chart
c. Hyporeflexia in the lower extremities
d. Ataxic gait

462. While in the ICU, you are called to your patient's bedside because of the development of seizure activity in a ventilator patient with nosocomial pneumonia. You review the situation including the medication record. The patient is currently receiving dopamine, one-half normal saline, imipenem/cilastatin, tobramycin, lisinopril, clonidine patch, and famotidine. The laboratory test results from this morning show normal electrolytes, except for a mildly elevated creatinine of 2.4 that is chronic, and CBC shows an improving white blood count of 15,000. After stopping the acute seizure event, you determine the next step in preventing further seizures is

a. Stop dopamine
b. Stop clonidine
c. Intravenous phenytoin
d. Change antibiotic coverage
e. CT of the head

463. Two days after admission, a 57-year-old man suddenly has a seizure. He was undergoing evaluation for substernal chest pain. The nursing staff noted that he seemed to be a little shaky since shortly after arrival on the floor. He has no history of seizures and a stat CT of the head performed during the postictal state was normal. Laboratory results had shown an MCV of 101 (elevated) and his AST was mildly elevated (one and one-half normal). In this patient, the most likely imbalance that would contribute to this event would be

a. Folate deficiency
b. Fasting hypoglycemia
c. Hypomagnesemia
d. Thiamine deficiency
e. Vitamin B_{12} deficiency

464. A 25-year-old man with a high-frequency fine tremor that may be difficult to see grossly has

a. Parkinson's disease
b. Essential tremor
c. Asterixis
d. Hyperthyroidism
e. Drug-related tremor

465. A 64-year-old man complains of a resting tremor that lessens with intentional movement and that causes him substantial embarrassment. What is the likely cause?

a. Parkinson's disease
b. Essential tremor
c. Asterixis
d. Hyperthyroidism
e. Drug-related tremor

466. The tremor associated with hepatic encephalopathy is

a. Resting tremor
b. Essential tremor
c. Asterixis
d. Very high frequency
e. Drug related

467. The tremor of which condition lessens with consumption of small amounts of alcohol

a. Parkinson's disease
b. Essential tremor
c. Asterixis
d. Hyperthyroidism
e. Drug-related tremor

468. A 65-year-old woman is seen for evaluation of dementia. On examination, you note that her left pupil does not react well to light. When she follows your finger with her eyes, as you approach the bridge of her nose, you note the left pupil to constrict equally as well as the right one. The most important test to order at this point would be

a. Titer for Lyme disease
b. B_{12} level
c. RPR
d. HIV
e. Fasting glucose

469. Which of the following muscle diseases with weakness is an autoimmune disorder?

a. Becker muscular dystrophy
b. Myotonic dystrophy
c. Glycogen storage disorder (acid maltase deficiency)
d. Duchenne muscular dystrophy
e. Myasthenia gravis

470. A 68-year-old man comes to your office with a complaint of right-sided jaw pain that occurs about half way through his meal. He has seen his dentist already and no abnormality was found. X-rays of the area were taken and they also were unremarkable. The next step in his workup should be

a. CT of the region
b. CBC
c. ESR
d. Calcium level
e. Carotid duplex

471. Which statement is true regarding the optic neuropathy that occurs with combined use of cigarettes and alcohol?

a. It is reversible with B vitamin supplements and abstinence
b. Color vision is not impaired
c. It is of sudden onset
d. Scotomas are present centrally

472. Entrapment of the median nerve causing carpal tunnel syndrome and if severe, muscle wasting in the thenar eminence of the hand, is associated with which of the following diseases?

a. Hypothyroidism
b. Diabetes
c. Amyloidosis
d. Rheumatoid arthritis
e. All of the above

473. A 75-year-old man is brought to your office by his son with concerns over developing dementia problems. Previously, the patient had been well and was forced to retire from his job a few months ago because of worsening arthritis symptoms limiting his mobility. He has been a widower for 7 months and he lives alone. His family is worried about his safety in view of these changes. The likely cause of this dementia picture is

a. HIV related
b. B_{12} deficiency
c. Depression
d. Multi-infarct dementia

474. A 35-year-old woman comes to your office complaining of weakness in her limbs and fatigability of her muscles, which, it seems to her, lessens after she rests. Sometimes she does not have any muscle weakness, for months at a time, and then she does; all this has been happening to her for the past few years. She tells you that what bothers her most is the "droopiness" of her eyelids. Which one procedure provides definitive confirmation of the diagnosis?

a. Single-fiber electromyography
b. CT scan or MRI of the head
c. Antiacetylcholine receptor radioimmunoassay
d. Edrophonium chloride test
e. Electroencephalogram (EEG)

475. A 38-year-old man presents to the emergency room with the sudden onset of a severe headache while chopping wood. This is the worst pain he has ever experienced, and it is accompanied by photophobia and vomiting. Which procedure(s) provide the best chance of making the diagnosis?

a. CT scan of the head
b. Lumbar puncture
c. CT scan of the head and lumbar puncture
d. ECG, lumbar puncture, and x-rays of the skull
e. Pneumoencephalogram

476. Excitatory neurotransmitters such as acetylcholine and glutamate perform which of the following functions?

a. Open cation channels and allow influx of Na^+ or Ca^{++}.
b. Generate inhibitory postsynaptic potentials
c. Activate mitochondria
d. Regulate intracellular K^+
e. Carry impulses between peripheral nerves only

477. A 25-year-old graduate student is injured in a fall during a weekend rock climbing expedition. There is serious damage to the peripheral nerves in his leg. Which of the following can be expected to occur?

a. Denervated muscles will hypertrophy
b. Individual muscle fibers will not be able to contract spontaneously
c. Groups of muscle fibers will not be able to spontaneously discharge
d. Normal motor function may never return
e. Muscle bulk may increase by one-half within 2 to 3 months

478. Weakness is caused by diseased anterior horn cells in which of the following disorders?

a. Myasthenia gravis
b. Botulism
c. Amyotrophic lateral sclerosis
d. Aminoglycoside antibiotic–associated weakness
e. Lambert-Eaton myasthenic syndrome

479. A 45-year-old man who has consumed excess alcohol for at least 20 years is seen for evaluation of progressive difficulty in walking. He has an ataxic gait and his muscles are generally hypotonic. He has an intention tremor in his arms and legs and he also demonstrates "past pointing." His primary brain pathology will be found in the

a. Occipital cortex
b. Temporal lobe
c. Cerebellum
d. Brainstem
e. Frontal cortex

480. A patient who has been diabetic for 15 years comes to your office complaining of a burning or tingling sensation in both of his feet and the lower aspects of both legs, which bothers him especially at night. His most likely diagnosis is

a. Mononeuropathy
b. Brown-Séquard's syndrome
c. Polyneuropathy
d. Mononeuropathy multiplex
e. Radiculopathy

481. A moderately obese factory worker who stands for long periods of time begins to experience pain and a severe burning sensation that is localized over the left anterior lateral thigh. This patient has a

a. Mononeuropathy
b. Brown-Séquard's syndrome
c. Polyneuropathy
d. Mononeuropathy multiplex
e. Radiculopathy

482. A man who was stabbed in the back during a fight is brought to the emergency room. On examination you find impaired pain and temperature sensation in one leg and impaired proprioception and vibration sense in the opposite leg. These findings are descriptive of a

a. Mononeuropathy
b. Brown-Séquard's syndrome
c. Polyneuropathy
d. Mononeuropathy multiplex
e. Radiculopathy

483. A 38-year-old woman with rheumatoid arthritis develops worse joint pain and also pain and paresthesias in scattered locations in both arms and both legs. Her sedimentation rate increases significantly and you diagnose vasculitis causing

a. Mononeuropathy
b. Brown-Séquard's syndrome
c. Polyneuropathy
d. Mononeuropathy multiplex
e. Radiculopathy

484. A 55-year-old man who has worked for many years as a stevedore develops pain and weakness in the lower back that radiates down the posterolateral thigh and lower aspect of the leg. This is characterized as

a. Mononeuropathy
b. Brown-Séquard's syndrome
c. Polyneuropathy
d. Mononeuropathy multiplex
e. Radiculopathy

485. An amenorrheic 35-year-old woman with galactorrhea is found to have a large prolactin-secreting pituitary tumor compressing her optic chiasm. Which visual disturbance does she have?

a. Left central scotoma
b. Bitemporal hemianopsia
c. Left nasal hemianopsia
d. Left homonymous hemianopsia
e. Completely blind left eye

486. A 2-year-old boy is brought to your office by his parents who believe he may not have normal hearing. You determine that he has congenital damage to the left cochlea. This is classified as a kind of

a. Conductive deafness
b. Sensorineural deafness
c. Central deafness
d. Tinnitus
e. Presbycusis

487. A 77-year-old man complains to you of an annoying buzzing sound in his right ear that bothers him mostly at night. This is classified as

a. Conductive deafness
b. Sensorineural deafness
c. Central deafness
d. Tinnitus
e. Presbycusis

488. Deafness due to disease of the cochlear nuclei or auditory pathways is classified as

a. Conductive deafness
b. Sensorineural deafness
c. Central deafness
d. Tinnitus
e. Presbycusis

489. A teenage girl presents for evaluation of hearing loss in her right ear. She has a history of at least 12 episodes of otitis media as a child; at least one time she perforated her ear drum. Her hearing loss is classified as

a. Conductive deafness
b. Sensorineural deafness
c. Central deafness
d. Tinnitus
e. Presbycusis

490. Which of the following clinical diagnoses is most often accompanied by coma?

a. Transient ischemic strokes
b. Creutzfeldt-Jakob disease or multi-infarct dementia
c. Cerebral hemorrhage, either subarachnoid or intracerebral
d. Amyotrophic lateral sclerosis
e. Small lacunar infarcts

491. Patients commonly complain of "dizziness." This symptom is

a. A well-defined sensation of one's environment spinning around
b. Usually accompanied by the physical finding of nystagmus
c. Usually accompanied by hearing loss
d. A loosely defined and nonspecific symptom of light-headedness or weakness or spinning
e. A specific sign of impending stroke

492. A 70-year-old man is brought to the ER because of sudden onset of right arm weakness and inability to understand speech. This speech problem is called

a. Apraxia
b. Aphasia
c. Abulia
d. Anomia
e. Alexia

493. A patient whom you have diagnosed with Alzheimer's disease is increasingly unable to retrieve from memory or to appropriately use previously learned words. This disorder is called

a. Apraxia
b. Aphasia
c. Abulia
d. Anomia
e. Alexia

494. A 50-year-old man who is an alcoholic is severely injured in a barroom brawl. He sustains a major injury to the frontal lobes of his brain. Subsequently, he always seems apathetic and unemotional. This disorder is called

a. Apraxia
b. Aphasia
c. Abulia
d. Anomia
e. Alexia

495. The inability to read printed words is known as

a. Apraxia
b. Aphasia
c. Abulia
d. Anomia
e. Alexia

496. A 30-year-old woman undergoes surgery for a very large, but fortunately benign, brain tumor. For 2 days after the surgery she is unable to perform certain previously learned motor functions. This disorder is called

a. Apraxia
b. Aphasia
c. Abulia
d. Anomia
e. Alexia

497. Abnormalities in the cytosolic copper-zinc superoxide dismutase (SOD1) gene on chromosome 21 have been identified as factors in the pathophysiology of which degenerative disorder?

a. Parkinson's disease
b. Amyotrophic lateral sclerosis
c. Huntington's chorea
d. Alzheimer's Disease
e. Tuberous sclerosis

498. An 8-year-old girl is noted to be having frequent "staring" spells during which she seems oblivious to her surroundings. She seems to suddenly return to awareness without realizing that she has been temporarily "out." The most likely finding on a full evaluation would be

a. Three per second (3-Hz) spike and wave activity on EEG
b. Abnormal reflexes in her lower extremities
c. An abnormal CT scan showing an occipital mass
d. An abnormal MRI showing demyelination
e. An abnormal mental status examination showing disorientation to time

499. Which clinical scenario best describes a patient with midstage dementia of the Alzheimer's type?

a. A patient has gradually developed memory deficits over the past four or five years; the deficits worsen each time he has a "spell," described by the family as "little strokes that get better in a few days"
b. A patient has had Parkinson's disease for years, and after becoming nearly immobile, he is also noted to have memory and language deficits
c. A patient has become progressively more withdrawn and shows deficits in short- and long-term memory; these deficits have been noticed by the family since the patient's wife and his last sibling died about 5 months ago
d. A patient became socially withdrawn a couple of years ago because he could not keep up with his friends' activities such as golf and bridge; now he is getting lost whenever he leaves his house
e. A long-term, often homeless, alcoholic becomes progressively disoriented and confused, and the condition cannot be reversed by a move to a nursing home where he receives adequate nutrition and medical care

500. Which cerebral artery is blocked in an ischemic stroke that presents with the following symptoms: aphasia, right hemiparesis, and right arm numbness?

a. Right anterior cerebral
b. Right middle cerebral
c. Right proximal posterior cerebral
d. Left anterior cerebral
e. Left middle cerebral

Nervous System

Answers

456. The answer is c. *(Fauci, 14/e, p 2533.)* This is the classic presentation of carbon monoxide poisoning, which includes confusion, shortness of breath, tachycardia, and reddish appearance of the mucous membranes. There would be a discrepancy between the pO_2 and O_2 saturation on the ABG. Pulse oximetry would be correct in the O_2 saturation estimation.

457. The answer is d. *(Fauci, 14/e, pp 559, 160; Adams, p 470.)* Although all of these processes may cause Horner's syndrome, the most common cause remains idiopathic. The Pancoast tumor and dissection of the carotid impinge on the sympathetic nerves, thus exerting their effect. Brainstem strokes would work at the central level to interrupt the sympathetic nerves.

458. The answer is d. *(Fauci, 14/e, p 77.)* This syndrome is called pseudoclaudication. It may also occur at times with exertion, thus causing confusion with peripheral vascular disease. Nerve impingement by osteoarthritis and by degenerative disk disease tends to give a radicular pattern to the discomfort.

459. The answer is d. *(Fauci, 14/e, pp 71, 1917–1918.)* There is a high correlation between temporal arteritis and the occurrence of polymyalgia rheumatica, and this would explain the proximal muscle girdle pain that is a frequent finding in temporal arteritis. This disease is an inflammation of the small arteries although there may be some involvement of the middle-sized arteries. The only laboratory test to attempt to confirm your diagnosis is to obtain an ESR, which should be elevated above 100. Definitive diagnosis is by temporal artery biopsy. Treatment with steroids prevents the occurrence of blindness as a complication. The elevated level of alkaline phosphatase is an incidental finding, perhaps because of alcohol consumption.

460. The answer is b. *(Fauci, 14/e, p 160.)* This disorder is benign and generally noted in younger females where it is felt to represent a mild dysautonomia. Tonic pupils may be seen also in diabetes, segmental hypo-hidrosis, Shy-Drager hyperhidrosis syndrome and amyloidosis.

461. The answer is c. *(Fauci, 14/e, p 160.)* Hyporeflexia in the lower extremities may be seen with this benign condition.

462. The answer is d. *(Fauci, 14/e, p 865.)* β-Lactam antibiotics, in particular high-dose penicillin G and imipenin, are known to induce seizures especially in the face of renal dysfunction. Acute treatment of the seizure would be the same as for any other source of seizure. Other medications could contribute to lowering seizure threshold via lowering the magnesium level (such as diuretics). The use of phenytoin should not be necessary unless recurrent events occur. The CT of the head is reasonable; however, the discontinuation of the β-lactam would be the first step.

463. The answer is c. *(Fauci, 14/e, pp 2265, 2504–2505.)* Alcohol withdrawal seizures are suspected because the man became shaky 2 days after admission in the hospital where he would not have access to alcoholic beverages, he has a macrocytosis consistent with folate deficiency due to alcoholism, and the diagnostic tests showed no underlying neurologic disease. The consumption of alcohol leads to excessive loss of magnesium in the urine and thus lowers seizure threshold. The AST level in general will increase more in the face of alcohol usage than will the ALT. The bulk of alcohol withdrawal seizures will occur within 5 days of the cessation of alcohol consumption.

464. The answer is d. *(Fauci, 14/e, pp 113–114, 424t, 1716.)* The tremor of hyperthyroidism is very high frequency and fine, unlike the tremors of Parkinsonism, asterixis, essential, and drug related. It does not depend on rest or movement. The tremor of Parkinson's disease is a coarse resting tremor that decreases with intentional movement. Cogwheel rigidity is also seen. In hepatic encephalopathy, the "flapping" tremor of asterixis is seen. Drug-related tremors are usually seen with β-2 agonists and methylxanthines. These are frequently of abrupt onset and time related to the usage or dosage adjustment with these medications.

465. The answer is a. *(Fauci, 14/e, pp 113–114, 424t, 1716.)* The tremor of Parkinson's disease is a coarse resting tremor that decreases with intentional movement. Cogwheel rigidity occurs in Parkinsonism. By contrast, the tremor of hyperthyroidism is very high frequency and fine, and it does not depend on rest or movement. In hepatic encephalopathy, the "flapping" tremor of asterixis is seen. Drug-related tremors are usually seen with β-2 agonists and methylxanthines. These are frequently of abrupt onset and time related to the usage or dosage adjustment with these medications.

466. The answer is c. *(Fauci, 14/e, pp 113–114, 424t, 1716.)* In hepatic encephalopathy, the "flapping" tremor of asterixis is seen. It can be elicited by gently extending the hand and holding it in that position. The other tremors are not elicited by these manipulations.

467. The answer is b. *(Fauci, 14/e, pp 113–114, 424t, 1716.)* An essential tremor lessens with small amounts alcohol consumption. The tremors of hyperthyroidism, Parkinson's disease, hepatic encephalopathy, and those related to drug ingestion do not do so.

468. The answer is c. *(Fauci, 14/e, p 160.)* This is the typical Argyll Robertson pupil found in syphilis. The RPR (rapid plasma reagin), a nontreponemal antibody test for syphilis, will be positive.

469. The answer is e. *(Fauci, 14/e, pp 2469–2479.)* Myasthenia gravis is an autoimmune disorder in which specific antibodies to acetylcholine receptors (AchRs) reduce the number of AChRs available at neuromuscular junctions. Becker muscular dystrophy and Duchenne muscular dystrophy (called pseudohypertrophic muscular dystrophy) are X-linked hereditary myopathies, and myotonic dystrophy is an autosomal dominant hereditary myopathy, all muscular dystrophies. Glycogen storage disorder is an autosomal recessive disorder with muscle weakness because of the acid maltase deficiency and glycogen accumulation; the adult form begins in the thirties or forties.

470. The answer is c. *(Fauci, 14/e, pp 1917–1918.)* Jaw claudication is a classic presentation of temporal arteritis. The ESR in this disease should be greater than 100 in general. The definitive diagnosis is by temporal artery biopsy only.

471. The answer is d. *(Fauci, 14/e, p 2457.)* The typical deficiency amblyopia that occurs with these substances is a gradual process with no reversibility; only stability of the current status can be achieved. Color vision may be affected and scotomas in the central or paracentral location are common.

472. The answer is e. *(Fauci, 14/e, pp 2466, 1933–1934.)* Carpal tunnel syndrome is typically associated with repetitive use of the hand/forearm, and multiple diseases may contribute also including these. Pregnancy may also cause this condition to surface; however, in this situation, it generally improves postpartum.

473. The answer is c. *(McPhee, 2/e, p 156; Fauci, 14/e, p 147.)* As many as 10 to 15% of patients evaluated for dementia are found to have depression. Care must be taken not to overlook this diagnosis as the underlying cause of dementia or an aggravating factor. Severe depression affecting multiple areas of life are seen commonly with 6 to 9 months after the loss of a spouse.

474. The answer is c. *(Fauci, 14/e, pp 2469–2472.)* This woman likely has myasthenia gravis; the incidence in women peaks in their twenties and thirties and women are more often affected, about 3:2, than men. Measurement of the antibody antiacetylcholine receptor provides a definitive diagnosis in 90% of cases of generalized disease, which this patient manifests, and 50% in ocular disease alone. Single-fiber electromyography is not specific for myasthenia gravis. Edrophonium chloride test, if unequivocally positive, makes the diagnosis highly probable. CT scan, MRI scan, and the EEG do not play a role in the diagnosis of myasthenia gravis.

475. The answer is c. *(Fauci, 14/e, p 2345.)* This patient has symptoms and signs consistent with a subarachnoid hemorrhage (SAH), which is associated with berry aneurysm, AV malformations, cocaine use, and extension of primary intracerebral hemorrhage and is reported to occur in conjunction with exertion. Typically, episodes of SAH begin suddenly and are severe in nature. The patient usually comments that "its the worst headache I've ever had." The lack of objective neurologic findings is common. The severity of the episode and the presence of vomiting along with loss of consciousness 50% of the time suggests this diagnosis. The CT will miss 20% of these hemorrhages and a lumbar puncture (LP) is required to completely exclude this diagnosis. A lumbar puncture can show the presence of subarachnoid blood. The ECG may have a prolongation of the QRS complex, prolongation of the QT interval or T wave changes consisting of inversions or tall peaked waves. However, skull x-rays or pneumoencephalogram do not aid in the diagnosis.

476. The answer is a. *(McPhee, 2/e, p 126.)* Excitatory neurotransmitters generate excitatory postsynaptic potentials by opening channels that allow Na^+ and Ca^{++} to enter neurons. Different neurotransmitters, such as GABA and glycine, cause inhibition of signals.

477. The answer is d. *(McPhee, 2/e, p 131.)* Fasciculation, fibrillation, and substantial atrophy can be expected. Normal muscle function will not likely return without aggressive medical intervention and may not return at all.

478. The answer is c. *(McPhee, 2/e, pp 130, 149; Fauci, 14/e, pp 2368, 2469–2472.)* The weakness of ALS ("Lou Gehrig's disease") is due to diseased motor neurons in the anterior horn cells. The weakness in the other disorders is caused by impaired neuromuscular transmission—by impaired calcium channel function in aminoglycoside-associated weakness, by autobodies to the calcium channels in Lambert-Eaton syndrome, by toxins that prevent neurotransmitter release in botulism, and by autobodies to neurotransmitter receptors in myasthenia gravis.

479. The answer is c. *(McPhee, 2/e, p 134; Fauci, 14/e, p 116.)* The cerebellum functions as a coordinating center for the maintenance of muscle tone and the regulation of motor tasks. It does not supply nerve impulses to directly cause muscles to contract.

480–484. The answers are 480: c; 481: a; 482: b; 483: d; 484: e. *(McPhee, 2/e, p. 140; Fauci, 14/e, pp 2460–2468.)* Numerous localized disorders and many systemic diseases can damage the spinal cord or the peripheral nerves. The pattern of pain, sensory loss, and sometimes weakness can help classify the disorder. A mononeuropathy involves pain/temperature and vibratory/joint position abnormalities, along the precise path of an individual nerve with associated weakness and pain. Mononeuropathy multiplex involves multiple noncontiguous peripheral nerves in a sequential fashion taking place over days to years. A radiculopathy involves a nerve root with dermatome distribution of both pain/temperature and vibratory/joint position abnormalities and weakness of the innervated muscles. Brown-Séquard's syndrome also involves pain/temperature and vibratory/joint position abnormalities; however, the distribution is ipsilateral pain/temperature and contralateral vibratory/joint position abnormalities with an ipsilateral motor deficit. A polyneuropathy similarly involves pain/temperature and vibratory/joint position abnormalities with a stocking-glove distribution and painful paraesthesias.

485. The answer is b. (*McPhee, 2/e, p 142; Fauci, 14/e, pp 161–163, 1974–1975.*) The optic chiasm is the area where fibers receiving input from both temporal visual fields cross. Compression at the chiasm causes dysfunction in both sets of fibers and thus loss of vision in both temporal visual fields.

486–489. The answers are 486: b; 487: d; 488: c; 489: a. (*McPhee, 2/e, p 145; Fauci, 14/e, pp 175–179.*) Sounds must be conducted through the middle ear and sensed by the cochlea and CN VIII; then they are processed by the cochlear nuclei and CNS pathways. Conductive deafness is hearing loss due to external auditory canal or middle ear disease. Sensineural deafness is a perceptive loss of hearing due to disease of the inner ear or eighth nerve. In conductive deafness, bone conduction is better than air conduction, and the reverse is the case for sensineural deafness. Central deafness is caused by disease affecting the central auditory pathways. Tinnitus an annoying noise in the ear that is usually benign, often is caused by cochlear or eighth nerve disorders. Hearing may be diminished, but the patient is not rendered fully deaf. Presbyacusis is hearing loss due to advanced age.

490. The answer is c. (*McPhee, 2/e, pp 147–148; Fauci, 14/e, pp 125–134.*) Many toxins and metabolic disturbances cause coma, as do structural lesions such as hemorrhages and large infarcts. Dementing illnesses do not ordinarily cause coma, although in their terminal stages, patients may be bedridden and virtually unresponsive.

491. The answer is d. (*McPhee, 2/e, p 146; Fauci, 14/e, pp 100–107.*) Dizziness is a nonspecific term and an ill-defined symptom sometimes describing faintness or weakness and sometimes meaning true vertigo. "Vertigo" should be used only when there is actually a sensation of movement; usually, the patient feels that he or she is spinning or the room is spinning around them.

492–496. The answers are 492: b; 493: d; 494: c; 495: e; 496: a. (*McPhee, 2/e, p 148; Fauci, 14/e, pp 134–142.*) Although various areas of the cerebral cortex are specialized to perform certain functions, the cognitive and behavioral domains (language, memory, calculation ability, and so forth) are interconnected to both cortical and subcortical neural networks. Specific deficits identified in a careful neurologic exam will help define which area or network has been damaged. Aphasia is an abnormality of language. Anomia, the inability to name, is a form of aphasia. Apraxia is a complex motor deficit not attributable to pyramidal, extrapyramidal, cerebellar, or sensory abnormalities.

497. The answer is b. (*McPhee, 2/e, pp 150–151.*) Abnormalities in the SOD1 gene have been linked to amyotrophic lateral sclerosis (ALS; Lou Gehrig's disease). The intact SOD1 gene catalyzes the formation of hydrogen peroxide from superoxide anion; the hydrogen peroxide is detoxified by catalase to form water. The mutant gene in some forms of ALS catalyzes the reduction of hydrogen peroxide to hydroxyl radicals which may contribute to the pathogenesis of ALS.

498. The answer is a. (*McPhee, 2/e, pp 154–155. Fauci, 14/e, pp 2311–2324.*) The EEG abnormality described is typical of "absence" seizures. This disorder typically presents with the clinical scenario described in this question.

499. The answer is d. (*McPhee, 2/e, pp 155–158; Fauci, 14/e, pp 2348–2353.*) "A" describes a patient with probable multi-infarct dementia; "B" is a patient with "Parkinson's dementia complex" or perhaps Lewy body disease; "C" is consistent with the pseudodementia of depression. "D" is the description most closely associated with Alzheimer's disease although the student should realize that the clinical syndromes may overlap considerably. Case "E" describes a long-term alcoholic whose dementia may be multifactorial, with possible direct toxic damage to the brain, possible nutritional deficits, and a social history that might well include episodes of head trauma.

500. The answer is e. *(McPhee, 2/e, p 160; Fauci, 14/e, pp 2328–2336.)* An infarction of the left hemisphere causes weakness or paralysis and sensory loss on the right. Most right-handed patients have their dominant speech center on the left, and it is supplied by the middle cerebral artery, as is the somatic motor area.

Bibliography

Barron WM, Lindheimer MD: *Medical Disorders During Pregnancy,* 2/e. St. Louis, Mosby, 1995.

Fauci AS, Braunwald E, Isselbacher KJ, Wilson JD, Martin JB, Kasper DL, Hauser SL, Longo DL (eds): *Harrison's Principles of Internal Medicine,* 14/e. New York, McGraw-Hill, 1998.

Lilly LS (ed): *Pathophysiology of Heart Disease.* Philadelphia, Lea & Febiger, 1993.

McPhee SJ, Lingappa VR, Ganong WF, Lange JD (eds): *Pathophysiology of Disease,* 2/e. Stamford, Connecticut, Appleton & Lange, 1997.

Murray PR, Rosenthal KS, Kobayashi GS, Pfaller MA: *Medical Microbiology,* 5/e. St. Louis, Mosby, 1997.

Roitt R, Brolstoff J, Male D: *Immunology,* 5/e. London, Mosby International, 1998.

Index